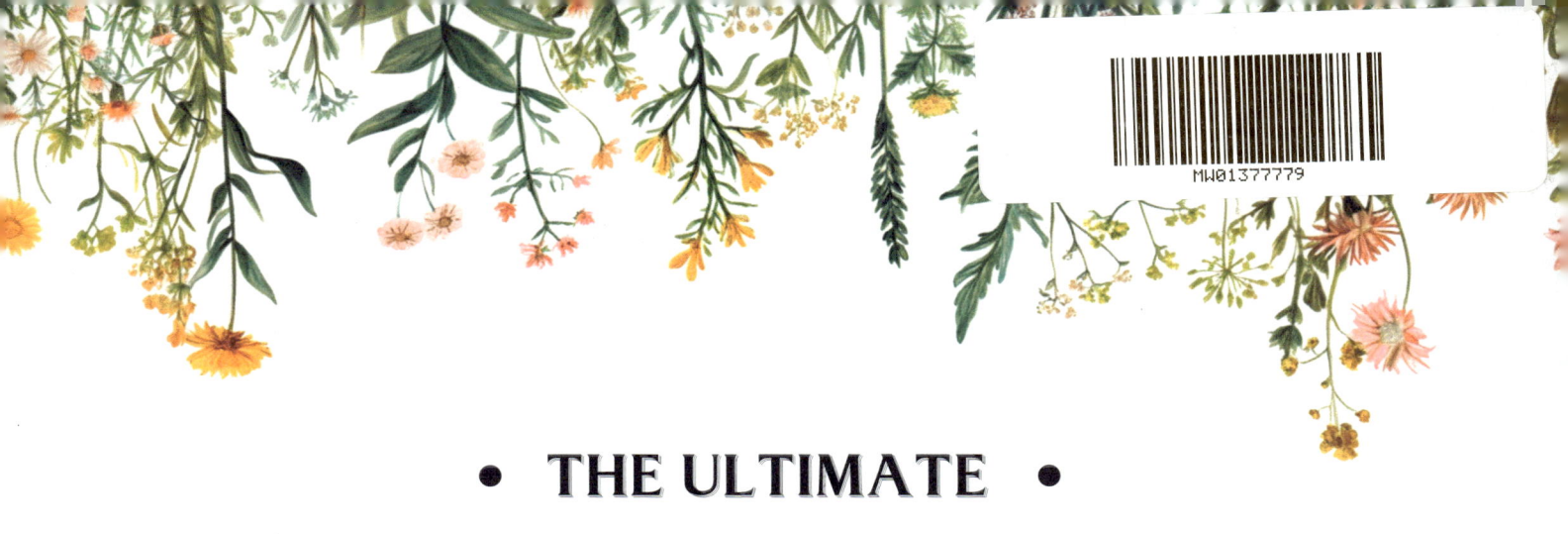

• THE ULTIMATE •

HOME
APOTHECARY

Powerful Time-Tested Remedies to Heal, Soothe, and Energize

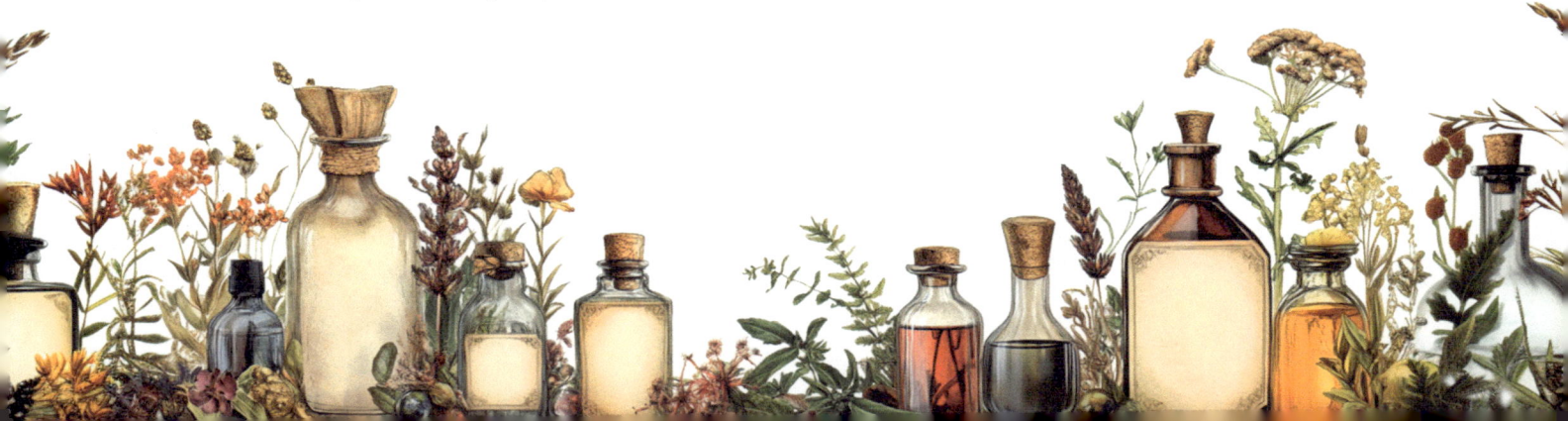

Table of Contents

Disclaimer 4

Introduction 5

Skin Problems and Wounds 6
1. Herbal Drawing Salve for Skin Irritations 7
2. Chickweed & Vinegar Soothing Skin Bath.................7
3. Antibacterial Healing Cream 8
4. Calendula & Comfrey Healing Blend 8
5. Yarrow Hemostatic Powder 9
6. Lavender Skin Healing Oil 9
7. Chamomile Scar Soothing Lotion 10
8. Soothing Honey & Oat Eczema Soap Bar 10
9. Psoriasis Relief Herbal Salve 11
10. Arnica & Calendula Healing Mist 11
11. Cooling Herbal Burn Relief Gel 12
12. Natural Bug Off Spray 12
13. Anti-Mosquito Salve 13
14. Plantain & Coconut Itch Relief Balm 13
15. Antiseptic Ointment 14
16. Herbal Wound Care Elixir 14

Personal Care 15
1. Herbal Hair Growth Tonic.................................. 16
2. Age Spot Rejuvenation Balm 16
3. Herbal Fresh Mint Toothpaste 17
4. Herbal Gum Care Mouthwash 17
5. Natural Youth Elixir 18
6. Glow & Balance Face Elixir 18
7. Herbal Breeze Natural Deodorant...................... 19
8. Herbal Sun Protect Lotion 19

Endocrine System...20
1. Nature's PCOS Aid 21
2. Pancreas Support Spiced Milk 21
3. Blood Sugar Balance Tea 22
5. Rhodiola Stress Relief Capsules 22
6. Pancreas Health Herbal Blend 23
7. Hormonal Harmony Tea 23
8. Gut Soother Infusion 24
9. Bladderwrack Tincture for Thyroid Support 24

Digestive System 25
1. Black Milk... 26
2. Gut Soother Infusion 26
3. Gut Detox Herbal Flush 27
4. Fermented Cabbage Elixir (Best Probiotic) 27
5. Natural Yarrow Bloat Extract 28
6. Hemorrhoid Soothing Elixir 28
7. Soothing Digestive Kombucha........................... 29
8. 4-Ingredient Digestive Elixir 29
9. Peaceful Night Infusion 30
10. Upset Stomach Comfort Syrup.......................... 30
11. Lemon and Ginger Nausea Lollipops 31
12. Restorative Liver Tea 31
13. Fatty Liver Tincture.. 32
14. Moringa Powder for Liver Detox 32
15. Peppermint Ease for IBS 33
16. Dandelion & Gentian Digestive Tonic 33
17. Ginger & ACV for Bloating and Gas Relief 34

18. Dandelion Lemonade for Gallbladder Health 34
19. Rejuvelac for Digestive Wellness 34
20. Gut Health Morning Shots 35
21. Herbal Acid Reflux Reliever 35
22. Ulcer & Gastritis Relief Tea 36
23. Bowel Balance Elixir....................................... 36
24. Anti-Parasitic Black Walnut Drops 37
25. Nature's Laxative Blend 37
26. Homemade Colon Detox Shot 38

Detox **39**
1. Bay Leaf Water 40
2. Flat Tummy Capsules 40
3. Craving Buster Brew 41
4. Dandelion and Burdock Purge 41
5. Metabolic Herbal Coffee................................... 42
6. Green Burn Smoothie 42
7. Forskolin Capsules to Boost Metabolism............. 43
8. Cleansing Stinging Nettle Soup 43
9. Metabolic Superfood Bars................................ 44
10. All-Day Slimming Tea 44

Respiratory System **45**
1. Mullein and Marshmallow Cough Syrup 46
2. Rosemary and Sage Sore Throat Spray 46
3. Honey Lemon Ginger Cough Drops 47
4. Mustard Plaster 47
5. Heating Potato Pad 48
6. Amish Cough Syrup 48
7. Sinus Relief Eucalyptus Steam 49
8. Hot Herbal Compress for Sinus Infection Relief 49
9. Herbal Gargle for Throat Infection Relief............. 50
10. Soothing Elixir for Cold and Flu Relief................ 50
11. Grandma's Herbal Antibiotic 51
12. Homemade Rub for Easy Breathing 51
13. Breath-Ease Thyme Syrup 52
14. Lung Strength Drops 52
15. Frontier Cough Soother 53
16. Warm Comfort Brew 53
17. Jello Flu Shots 54
18. Clear Chest Basil Brew 54
19. Soothing Relief Balm 55
20. Allergy-Ease Herbal Tea................................. 55
21. Nettle Hay Fever Tincture 56
22. Mullein Mucus Buster 56
23. Onion Heat Relief Wrap 57
24. Cool Down Vinegar Wraps 57
25. Anti-Fever Elixir 58
26. Herbal Fever Compress.................................. 58
27. Snore Relief Jelly 59
28. Turmeric Tonic for Inflammation 59

Cardiovascular System **60**
1. Arterial De-Clogger 61
2. Warming Turmeric and Cayenne Balm to Promote Circulation...........61
3. Cinnamon Infusion for Blood Pressure 62
4. Heart Harmony Elixir with Hawthorn Berry 62
5. Garlic and Lemon Tonic for Cholesterol Management 63
6. Hibiscus Tea for Cardiovascular Support 63

7. Beetroot and Aronia Juice for Circulatory Health 64
8. Blood Vessel Care with Butcher's Broom 64
9. Bilberry Heart Drops.. 65
10. Horse Chestnut Cooling Gel for Varicose Veins 65
11. Young Heart Elixir 66

Nervous System **67**
1. Memory Elixir 68
2. Brain Boosting Tonic 68
3. Natural Brain Booster 69
4. Brain Power Mushroom Elixir 69
5. Mind Sharpening Infusion 70
6. Ginkgo Biloba Focus Fuel 70
7. Anti-Migraine Syrup 71
8. Herbal Blend for Headache Relief 71
9. Moon Milk for Better Sleep 72
10. Nature's Aspirin 72
11. Deep Sleep Banana Tea 73
12. Soothing Herbal Soak 73
13. St. John's Wort and Linden Calming Infusion 74
14. Nature's Sedative Home Apothecary 74
15. Stress-Free Elixir Home Apothecary..................... 75
16. Stress Relief Herbal Candle 75
17. At-Home Sedative to Alleviate Panic Attacks........... 76
18. Restorative Tablets to Ease Mental Pressure 76
19. "Sweet Dreams" Herbal Pillow 77
20. Herbal Sleeping Pills 77
21. Bath Salt Mix for Relaxation 78
22. Kava Extract to Unwind & Get Relief 78
23. The Legal Narcotic You Can Make at Home 79
24. Happiness Hormones Booster 79
25. Worry Relieving Tincture 80
26. Lemon Balm and Skullcap Relaxing Tisane 80
27. Peaceful Mind Drops 81

Auditory and Visual Systems **82**
1. Tinnitus Relief Glycerite 83
2. Vertigo Relief Herbal Infusion 83
3. Parsley Tinnitus Relief Patch............................. 84
4. Herbal Ear Relief Compress............................... 84
5. Natural Antibacterial Eye Drops 85
6. Soothing Calendula and Rose Eye Rinse................. 85
7. Cooling Cucumber and Aloe Eye Mask 86
8. Bilberry Vision Support Tonic 86
9. Ginkgo Biloba Vision & Circulation Boost Tincture 87
10. Eye-Guard Antioxidant Blend 87
11. Ear Relief Soothing Oil 88
12. Ear Comfort Relief Spray 88

Musculoskeletal Health **89**
1. Soothing Muscle & Joint Relief Balm..................... 90
2. Herbal Pain Relief Infusion................................ 90
3. Joint & Cartilage Soothing Balm 91
4. Comfrey & Lavender Muscle Relief Oil 91
5. Collagen Boosting Herbal Elixir 92
6. Sports Relief Herbal Liniment............................. 92
7. Grandma's Back Pain Relief Salve 93
8. Arthritis Relief Mobility Tincture 93
9. Natural Joint Pain Relief Remedy 94
10. Herbal Poultice for Arthritis Pain Relief 94
11. Herbal Anti-Inflammatory Tincture for Joint Relief.... 95
12. Soothing DIY Balm for Pain Relief and Skin Irritation 95
13. Pineapple & Turmeric Pain Relief Extract 96

14. Backyard Serenity Capsules 96
15. Magnesium Relief Cream for Leg Cramps 97
16. Fermented Red Clover Elixir for Bone Health 97
17. Soothe & Heal Dandelion Salve 98
18. Nourishing Watercress Bone Broth for Joint Health 98
19. Green Boost Juice for Bone Health 99
20. Cabbage Wraps for Joint Relief.......................... 99
21. Pine Needle Infusion for Joint and Muscle Relief........ 100
22. Willow Bark Soothing Soak for Pain and Inflammation .. 100
23. Herbal Pain-Relief Patch with Willow Bark and Turmeric ... 101
24. Fibromyalgia Soothing Herbal Tea Blend 101

Immune System **102**
1. Healing Penicillin Soup for Cold and Flu 103
2. Immune-Boosting Echinacea & Astragalus Tincture 103
3. Natural Immune Support Tea 104
4. Anti-Inflammatory Ginger & Turmeric Root Tea 104
5. Soothing Golden Turmeric & Ginger Salve 105
6. Homemade Cinchona Quinine Tonic 105
7. Nutrient-Dense Herbal Vitamin Snack Bars 106
8. Detoxifying Lymphatic Cleanser Tonic 106
9. Antiviral Mushroom Extract for Immune Support ... 107
10. Natural Butterfly Pea Tea for Immune Support 107
11. Immune Boosting White Cell Juice 108
12. Nature's Antibiotic Capsules 108
13. Amish Fire Cider 109
14. Blue Tea Bliss.. 109
15. Fungal Fighter Cream..................................... 110
16. Fungal Relief Salve 110
17. Natural Anti Wart Spray.................................. 111
18. Candida Relief Ointment.................................. 111
19. Viral Relief Oil 112
20. Herpes Comfort Balm 112
21. Heavy Metal Cleanse Powder............................ 113
22. Immune Soothing Mushroom Tincture 113
23. Elderberry Immunity Boost Syrup 114
24. Anti-Inflammatory Turmeric Milk 114
25. Immune-Boosting Herbal Honey 115

Reproductive System **116**
1. Hormonal Balance Menopause Elixir 117
2. Menstrual Relief Anise Seed Tea 117
3. Lunar Harmony Tea 118
4. Hormonal Balance & Skin Care Primrose Oil 118
5. Lactation Support Herbal Tea 119
6. Menstrual Comfort Herb Tincture 119
7. Fertility Support Tonic..................................... 120
8. Nature's Fertility Aphrodisiac 120
9. Male Vitality Herbal Tonic 121
10. Prostate Health Herbal Infusion......................... 121

Urinary System **122**
1. Soothing Corn Silk Tea 123
2. UTI-Fighting Herbal Tea Blend 123
3. Cranberry Hibiscus Detox Tea............................ 124
4. Parsley Detox & Urinary Health Tea 124
5. Kidney Cleanse Elixir 125
6. Kidney Detox Juice 125
7. Pumpkin Seed Bladder Support Tincture................ 126

Safety Guidelines **126**
1. Apothecary Care & Storage Tips 127
2. Proper Usage and Dosage 128
3. Side Effects and Allergies 128

Disclaimer

This book is intended to provide historical information about natural medicines, remedies, and cures used in the past. The publisher, editor, and authors do not provide legal or medical advice. If you are unwell or considering any remedies, always consult a qualified healthcare professional, such as your physician or another medical specialist.

This book does not claim to be comprehensive or exhaustive in its coverage of natural remedies. While every effort has been made to ensure the accuracy and usefulness of the content, typographical or factual errors may exist. As such, this book is not intended to serve as a medical guide.

The authors, editor, and publisher shall not be held liable for any loss, injury, or adverse effects—whether direct or indirect—resulting from the use of the information contained within. Any decision to use a remedy, tincture, decoction, or other preparation described in this book is undertaken at your own risk, and it is your responsibility to consult a medical professional before proceeding.

Certain remedies or practices mentioned may not comply with FDA guidelines. The information in this book has not been reviewed, tested, or approved by any official regulatory body.

The authors, editor, and publisher make no guarantees, expressed or implied, regarding the results of applying the information provided. Furthermore, they hold no responsibility for the misuse or misidentification of plants or any consequences to your health or that of others arising from such use.

Some names and identifying details have been changed to protect the privacy of individuals involved.

By continuing to read this book, you acknowledge and agree to this disclaimer. If you do not agree, you may return the book within the guarantee period for a full refund.

Introduction

Introduction to Home Apothecary Basics

Creating your own home apothecary is more than just a hobby; it's a step toward taking control of your wellness in a natural, empowered way. By crafting your own remedies, you're not only cutting down on unnecessary chemicals but also connecting with age-old traditions that value the healing power of nature. From calming teas to soothing salves, these remedies can become a practical, nurturing part of your everyday life.

Why It's Worth Creating Your Own Apothecary

When you make your own remedies, you know exactly what goes into each product and can tailor it to fit your unique needs. It's a creative, hands-on approach to self-care that aligns with a sustainable, mindful lifestyle. You'll save money by relying less on store-bought products and gain the satisfaction of knowing you're capable of managing minor ailments and boosting your well-being naturally.

Beyond the practical benefits, building a home apothecary is an investment in a healthier, more intentional lifestyle. With your own remedies at hand, you're prepared to handle daily discomforts without reaching for processed solutions. Plus, the practice of making remedies can be a calming ritual itself—a quiet, grounding break from the hustle of daily life.

The Benefits of Natural Remedies

Natural remedies have been used for centuries, drawing on the inherent properties of plants and herbs to address everything from digestive issues to stress relief. Unlike many synthetic alternatives, natural remedies work gently with your body. They can support long-term health without the side effects often found in pharmaceutical options. By incorporating these remedies into your lifestyle, you're giving your body access to the nutrients and compounds it recognizes and thrives on.

Essential Tools to Get Started

Building a home apothecary doesn't require an entire kitchen overhaul. With just a few essential tools, you can create everything from teas and tinctures to balms and poultices. Here's a list of some basics:

- **Glass Jars and Bottles:** Perfect for storing dried herbs, infused oils, and finished remedies. Choose airtight options to maintain freshness.

- **Mortar and Pestle:** Crush herbs and spices to release their natural oils and active compounds.

- **Double Boiler:** Useful for melting beeswax, shea butter, and oils without direct heat, preserving their potency.

- **Fine Mesh Strainer:** Helps in straining teas, tinctures, and oils to remove plant material and achieve a smooth consistency.

- **Measuring Spoons and Dropper Bottles:** For precise measurements, especially when working with essential oils or making tinctures.

- **Labels and Markers:** Always label your creations with the date and ingredients to keep track of freshness.

With these tools and a few simple ingredients, you'll be well on your way to crafting your own natural apothecary—a resource that's as rewarding to build as it is beneficial to use.

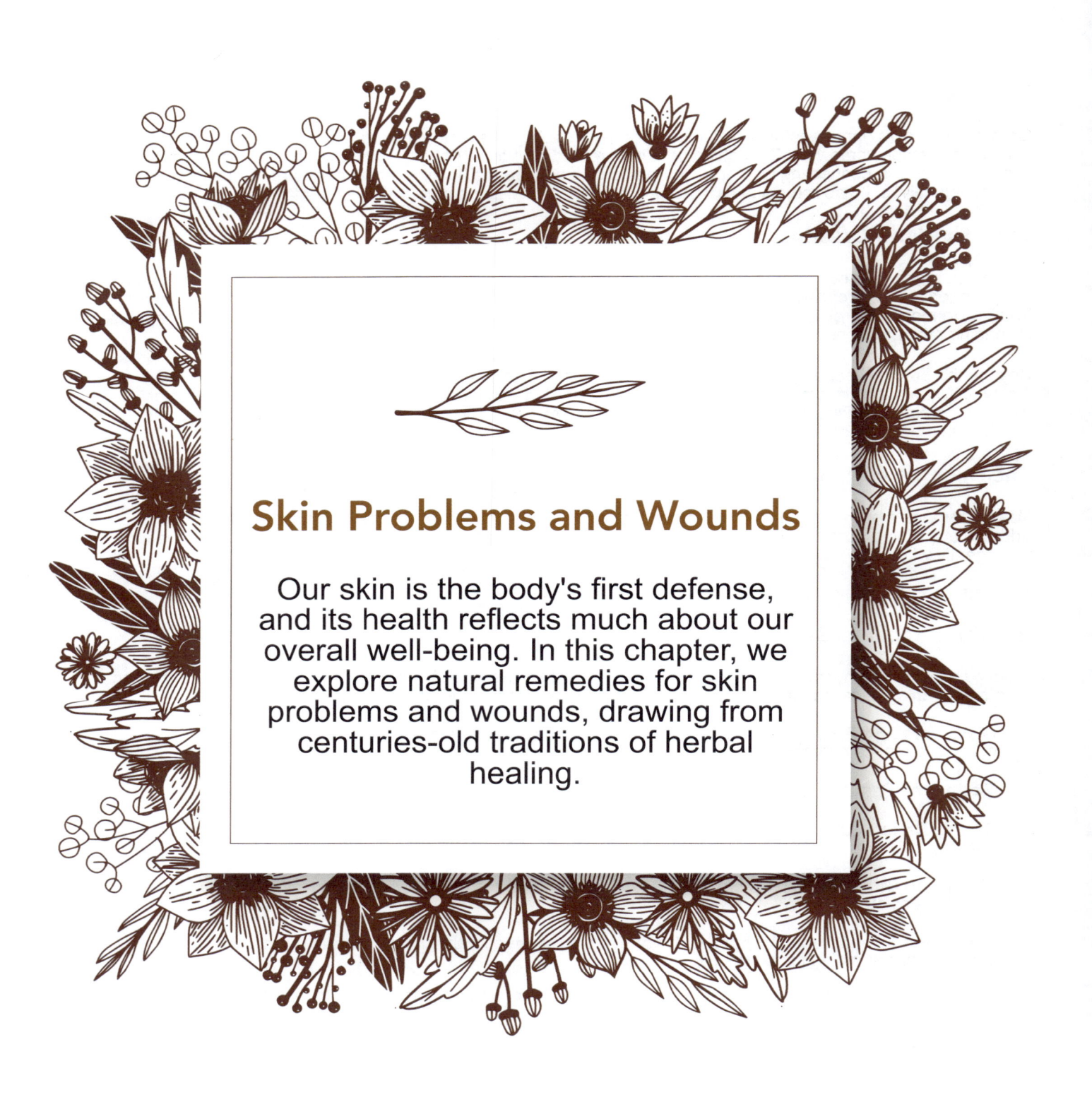

Skin Problems and Wounds

Our skin is the body's first defense, and its health reflects much about our overall well-being. In this chapter, we explore natural remedies for skin problems and wounds, drawing from centuries-old traditions of herbal healing.

Herbal Drawing Salve for Skin Irritations

This classic herbal remedy, often referred to as a black drawing salve, is used to draw out impurities, splinters, or ticks from the skin, as well as to help treat boils. Traditionally made with powerful natural ingredients, it has a history of use for aiding skin recovery and soothing irritation.

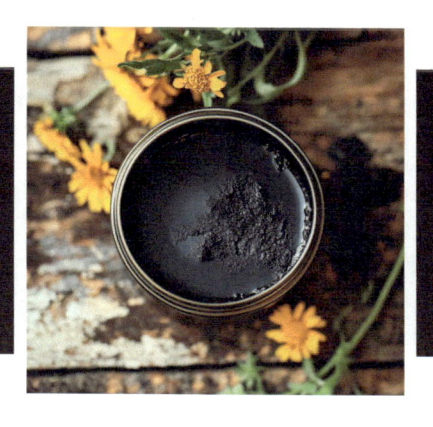

Ingredients:

- Activated Charcoal: Known for its toxin-binding properties, helps pull impurities.
- Bentonite Clay: Absorbs toxins and impurities, further enhancing the drawing effect.
- Beeswax: Provides a protective barrier on the skin, keeping the salve in place.
- Coconut Oil: Moisturizes and soothes irritated skin.
- Calendula Oil: Has skin-healing properties, helps reduce inflammation and soothe the area.

Instructions:

1. In a small saucepan over low heat, melt 1 tablespoon of beeswax with 2 tablespoons of coconut oil.
2. Add 1/2 teaspoon each of activated charcoal and bentonite clay, and mix thoroughly until smooth.
3. Remove from heat and stir in a few drops of calendula oil. Let the mixture cool slightly, then pour it into a clean container.
- Apply a small amount of the salve directly to the affected area, covering it with a bandage. Leave it on for several hours or overnight to allow the salve to draw out impurities. Reapply as needed until the issue is resolved.
- Store in a cool, dry place for up to six months.

Chickweed & Vinegar Soothing Skin Bath

This soothing bath combines the healing properties of chickweed with the natural cleansing effects of vinegar to ease skin rashes and irritation. Chickweed has been used traditionally to reduce inflammation and itching, while vinegar helps balance the skin's pH and can assist in soothing and cleaning affected areas.

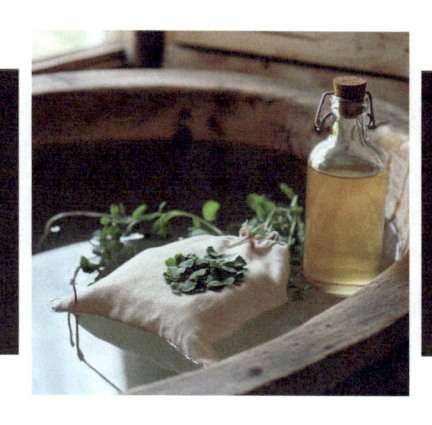

Ingredients:

- Chickweed (Stellaria media): Known for its anti-inflammatory, soothing, and healing properties, particularly for itchy, irritated skin.
- Apple Cider Vinegar: Balances skin pH and has mild antiseptic properties that can help cleanse the skin and reduce redness.
- Water: To dilute and make the bath comfortable and effective.

Instructions:

1. Fill a bathtub with warm water.
2. Add 1/4 cup of apple cider vinegar to the bath.
3. Place a handful of dried or fresh chickweed in a muslin bag or cheesecloth, tie it up, and place it in the water, letting it steep for 10–15 minutes.
4. Soak in the bath for 20–30 minutes, allowing the chickweed and vinegar to soothe your skin.
- Use this bath once or twice daily to relieve irritation from rashes, insect bites, or general skin inflammation. For best results, stay in the bath long enough for the skin to absorb the soothing properties of the herbs.
- Store any leftover chickweed infusion in the refrigerator for up to a few days to use for additional baths.

Antibacterial Healing Cream

This cream combines natural herbs known for their healing, antibacterial, and anti-inflammatory properties, offering a soothing treatment for minor cuts, scrapes, and skin infections. The combination of herbs like calendula, thyme, and lavender, along with the healing power of honey, helps fight bacteria while nourishing and regenerating the skin.

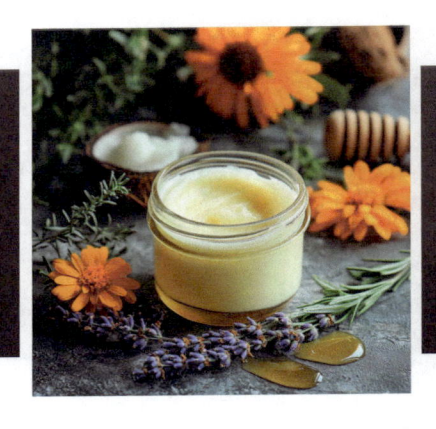

Ingredients:

- Calendula: Known for its skin-healing properties and ability to fight bacteria, calendula promotes faster wound healing and reduces inflammation.
- Thyme: A powerful antiseptic herb with natural antibacterial properties, thyme helps protect the skin from infection.
- Lavender: Offers soothing and antimicrobial benefits, helping to heal wounds and calm irritated skin.
- Honey: A natural humectant with antimicrobial properties, honey aids in wound healing and helps to maintain moisture in the skin.
- Coconut Oil: A nourishing oil that provides a base for the cream and helps with skin hydration.

Instructions:

1. In a double boiler, melt 1 tablespoon of beeswax along with 2 tablespoons of coconut oil until fully liquefied.
2. Once the mixture is melted, remove from heat and add 10 drops of tea tree oil, 5 drops of oregano oil, and 5 drops of lavender oil. Stir well to combine.
3. Allow the mixture to cool and solidify into a cream-like consistency.
4. Transfer the cream into a small glass jar for storage.
- Apply the herbal cream directly to the affected nail and surrounding skin twice daily.

Calendula & Comfrey Healing Blend

This soothing skin salve combines the healing properties of calendula and comfrey, two herbs long used for their ability to aid in the healing of wounds, cuts, and skin irritations. Calendula promotes tissue repair and reduces inflammation, while comfrey is known for its ability to speed up cell regeneration, making this salve an ideal remedy for treating dry skin, bruises, and minor cuts.

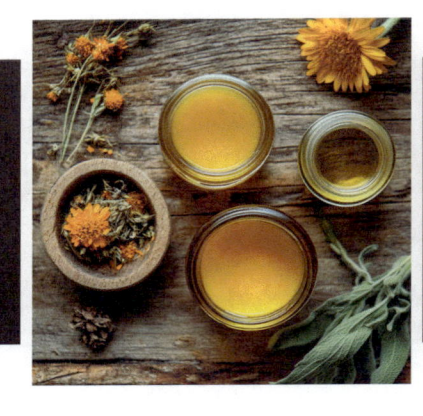

Ingredients:

- Calendula: Known for its anti-inflammatory and antiseptic properties, calendula helps to calm irritation, promote healing, and protect the skin.
- Comfrey: Contains allantoin, which supports skin cell regeneration and helps to speed up the healing process for wounds and injuries.
- Beeswax: A natural emulsifier that helps solidify the salve and provides a barrier to lock in moisture while protecting the skin.
- Coconut Oil: Nourishes and moisturizes the skin, serving as a base for the salve.
- Olive Oil: supports skin hydration and further boosts the salve's healing properties.

Instructions:

1. Infuse 1/4 cup of dried calendula and comfrey leaves in 1/2 cup of olive oil. Heat gently in a double boiler or saucepan for 30 minutes.
2. Strain the oil to remove the herbs, then return the oil to the heat.
3. Add 2 tablespoons of beeswax to the infused oil and stir until melted.
4. Remove from heat and stir in 2 tablespoons of coconut oil until fully combined.
5. Pour the mixture into small containers or tins and let it cool to set.
- Apply the salve to the affected area 2-3 times daily to soothe and promote healing of minor wounds, bruises, and skin irritations.

Yarrow Hemostatic Powder

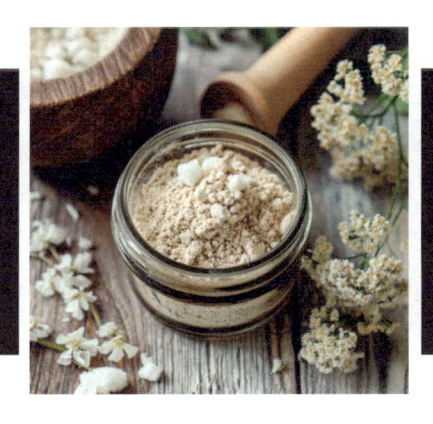

Yarrow is renowned for its ability to stop bleeding and promote healing. This simple but powerful herb has been used for centuries as a natural remedy for cuts, scrapes, and nosebleeds due to its astringent and hemostatic properties. The powder made from dried yarrow flowers can be applied directly to a wound to help control bleeding and aid in the healing process.

Ingredients:

- Dried Yarrow Flowers: Yarrow's astringent and styptic properties help to constrict blood vessels, stopping bleeding quickly.
- Optional: Marshmallow Root: Adds soothing properties, especially for irritated or inflamed skin.

Instructions:

1. Dry fresh yarrow flowers by hanging them upside down or using a dehydrator.
2. Once dried, crush the yarrow flowers into a fine powder using a mortar and pestle or grinder.
3. (Optional) Add a small amount of powdered marshmallow root to increase soothing effects.
4. Store the powder in an airtight container, away from light and moisture.
- When bleeding occurs, apply a small amount of yarrow powder directly to the wound and press gently. Hold in place until the bleeding stops. Reapply as needed. For deeper or more severe wounds, seek medical attention. Store powder in a cool, dry place, and it can last for several months.

Lavender Skin Healing Oil

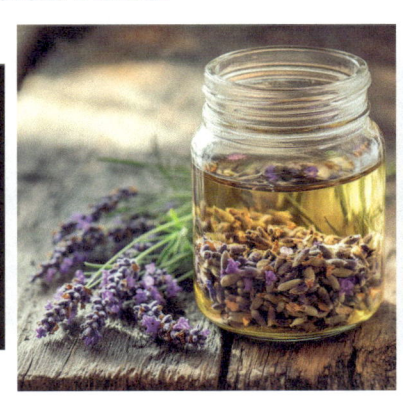

Lavender is widely known for its calming aroma, but its healing properties extend to the skin as well. Lavender-infused oil is commonly used for its regenerative effects on the skin, helping to reduce scars, promote healing, and alleviate irritation. This oil can be applied to minor cuts, burns, and even conditions like acne or eczema, thanks to its anti-inflammatory and antimicrobial properties.

Ingredients:

- Lavender Flowers: Known for their ability to calm inflammation and regenerate skin cells.
- Carrier Oil (Olive Oil, Jojoba Oil, or Sweet Almond Oil): Used as the base to infuse the lavender and allow for easy application on the skin.

Instructions:

1. Fill a clean glass jar halfway with dried lavender flowers.
2. Cover the flowers with your choice of carrier oil, ensuring they are fully submerged.
3. Seal the jar and store it in a warm, sunny spot for about 2-3 weeks. Shake the jar daily to help the infusion process.
4. After 2-3 weeks, strain the lavender flowers from the oil using a fine mesh strainer or cheesecloth.
5. Store the infused lavender oil in a clean, airtight container, away from direct sunlight.
- Apply a small amount of lavender-infused oil to affected areas of the skin once or twice a day. Gently massage it in and allow the oil to absorb. This oil can help promote healing for minor cuts, burns, or scars, and its soothing properties make it ideal for use on dry or irritated skin.

Chamomile Scar Soothing Lotion

Chamomile is known for its calming effects on the skin, ideal for reducing scars and supporting healing. Chamomile's anti-inflammatory and antioxidant properties make it effective in minimizing the appearance of scars while soothing the skin.

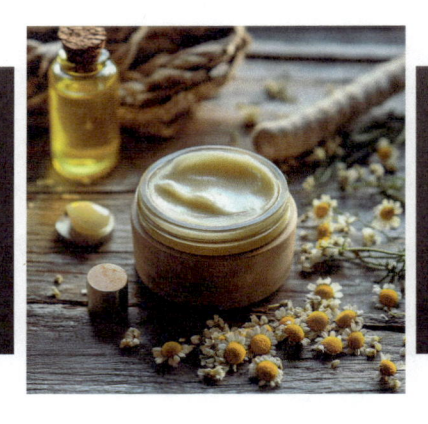

Ingredients:

- Dried Chamomile Flowers: Renowned for their soothing and healing effects, chamomile helps reduce redness and inflammation around scars.
- Olive Oil or Jojoba Oil: Nourishes and moisturizes the skin while aiding in the absorption of chamomile's beneficial compounds.
- Beeswax: Used to thicken the lotion and form a protective barrier on the skin.
- Vitamin E Oil: Acts as an antioxidant and helps promote skin healing.

Instructions:

1. Infuse Oil: In a double boiler, combine 1/4 cup dried chamomile flowers and 1/2 cup olive or jojoba oil. Heat on low for 30 minutes, stirring occasionally.
2. Strain: Remove from heat and strain out the flowers.
3. Blend: Heat the oil again on low, adding 1 tbsp beeswax until melted. Remove from heat and stir in a few drops of Vitamin E.
4. Cool and Store: Pour into a clean jar and let solidify.
5. Apply gently to scars once or twice daily for best results.

Soothing Honey & Oat Eczema Soap Bar

This honey oat soap blend is ideal for soothing and moisturizing sensitive skin, especially for those managing eczema and rashes. Honey and oats work together to ease inflammation, lock in moisture, and gently nourish the skin.

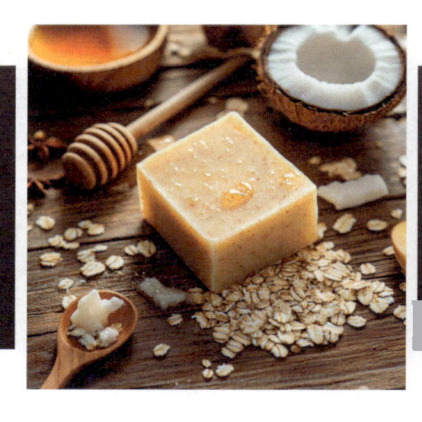

Ingredients:

- Colloidal Oatmeal: Ground oats help soothe irritation, reduce redness, and relieve itching.
- Honey: A natural humectant with antibacterial properties, honey helps to lock in moisture and heal inflamed skin.
- Olive Oil: A nourishing oil that gently hydrates and protects, ideal for sensitive skin.
- Coconut Oil: Provides a creamy lather and additional moisture to help ease dryness.
- Shea Butter: Rich in vitamins and fatty acids, shea butter helps soften and protect skin, preventing further irritation.

Instructions:

1. In a double boiler, melt olive oil, coconut oil, and shea butter together.
2. Once melted, remove from heat and stir in honey and colloidal oatmeal until well mixed.
3. Pour the mixture into soap molds.
4. Allow it to harden for about 24 hours.
5. After removing from molds, let the soap cure for at least two weeks to firm up.
- Use daily on affected skin areas during your bathing routine to soothe eczema and rashes. Store soap in a dry area between uses to prolong its lifespan and effectiveness.

Psoriasis Relief Herbal Salve

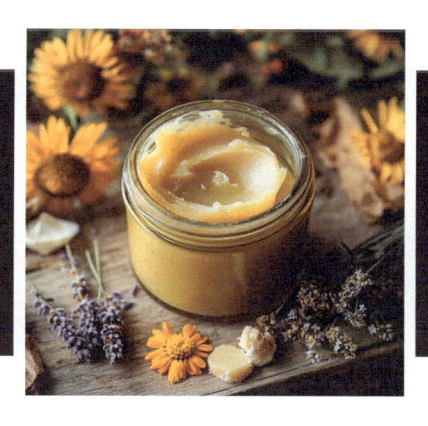

This herbal ointment provides soothing relief for psoriasis irritation, helping to calm inflammation and moisturize affected areas. The blend of herbs and oils in this ointment aims to alleviate itching and reduce the severity of flare-ups.

Ingredients:

- Calendula: 2 tablespoons (for anti-inflammatory and skin-soothing properties)
- Chamomile: 1 tablespoon (to reduce redness and irritation)
- Beeswax: 2 tablespoons (to create a protective barrier and lock in moisture)
- Olive Oil: 1/2 cup (to deeply moisturize and soften skin)
- Lavender Essential Oil: 5 drops (optional, for calming and added skin support)

Instructions:

1. In a double boiler, heat olive oil, calendula, and chamomile until herbs are thoroughly infused, about 30 minutes.
2. Strain the oil to remove herbs, and return to the double boiler.
3. Add beeswax and stir until fully melted and combined with the oil.
4. Remove from heat, and stir in lavender essential oil.
5. Pour into a clean container and allow it to cool and solidify.
- Apply a thin layer to psoriasis-affected areas as needed, particularly after bathing and before bed. Store in a cool, dry place for long-lasting relief.

Arnica & Calendula Healing Mist

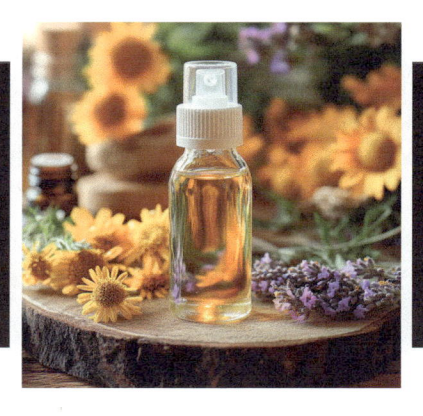

This natural first aid spray is designed to help soothe minor cuts, bruises, and skin irritations. Arnica and calendula are known for their skin-healing properties, making this spray ideal for a gentle, herbal approach to minor injuries.

Ingredients:

- Arnica Flowers: 1 tablespoon (helps reduce swelling and bruising)
- Calendula Oil: 1 tablespoon (promotes wound healing and reduces inflammation)
- Witch Hazel: 1/2 cup (as a natural astringent and skin cleanser)
- Distilled Water: 1/2 cup (dilutes and balances the formula)
- Lavender Essential Oil: 5-10 drops (optional, for added soothing effects)

Instructions:

1. In a small saucepan, combine distilled water and dried arnica and calendula flowers.
2. Bring to a gentle simmer, then remove from heat and let steep for 20 minutes.
3. Strain the mixture to remove the herbs, then pour the liquid into a clean spray bottle.
4. Add witch hazel and lavender essential oil (if using) to the bottle, and shake well to combine.
- Spray directly onto minor cuts, bruises, or skin irritations as needed. Allow the spray to dry on the skin for maximum effect. Store in a cool, dark place for up to a week for the best results.

Cooling Herbal Burn Relief Gel

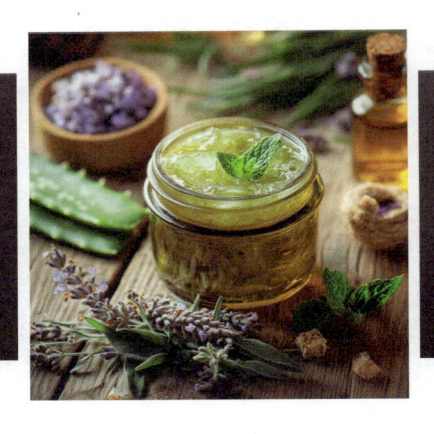

This soothing gel provides instant relief from minor burns by combining herbs known for their cooling and anti-inflammatory properties. Aloe vera, peppermint, and lavender work together to reduce pain and help promote skin repair.

Ingredients:

- Aloe Vera Gel: 1/4 cup (naturally cooling and promotes skin healing)
- Peppermint Essential Oil: 3-5 drops (offers cooling relief and reduces pain)
- Lavender Essential Oil: 5 drops (soothes and promotes skin repair)
- Calendula Oil: 1 teaspoon (optional, for additional anti-inflammatory support)

Instructions:

1. In a small bowl, combine aloe vera gel with peppermint and lavender essential oils.
2. Add calendula extract if using, and stir well to ensure all ingredients are blended.
3. Pour the mixture into a clean, airtight container.
- Apply a small amount of gel directly to the burn area. Repeat as needed to keep the skin moisturized and cool. Store in the refrigerator for added cooling relief.

Natural Bug Off Spray

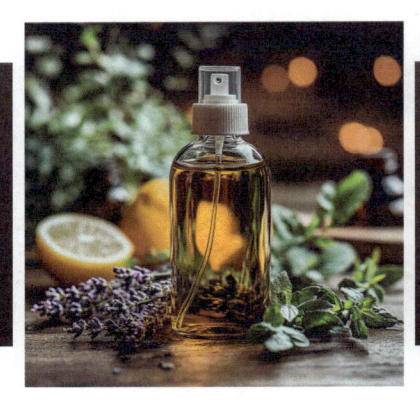

This natural bug repellent spray combines essential oils that are known for their ability to keep insects at bay. It's a safe and effective alternative to chemical-laden products, using ingredients that have long been trusted for their insect-repelling properties.

Ingredients:

- Witch Hazel: 1/2 cup (acts as the base and a gentle astringent)
- Tea Tree Essential Oil: 10 drops (has insect-repelling properties)
- Lavender Essential Oil: 10 drops (calming and also repels mosquitoes)
- Peppermint Essential Oil: 5 drops (repels mosquitoes and other insects)
- Lemon Eucalyptus Essential Oil: 10 drops (known for repelling mosquitoes)
- Water: 1/4 cup (to dilute and adjust the consistency)

Instructions:

1. In a spray bottle, combine the witch hazel and water.
2. Add the essential oils (lemon eucalyptus, tea tree, lavender, and peppermint).
3. Shake well to combine.
- Spray directly onto skin and exposed areas to deter insects. Reapply every few hours, especially after sweating or swimming. Shake the bottle before each use to ensure the oils mix properly.

Anti-Mosquito Salve

This natural anti-mosquito salve combines a selection of essential oils known for their insect-repellent properties, offering a safe, effective, and skin-friendly way to keep mosquitoes and other bugs at bay. It also moisturizes the skin, making it a great addition to your herbal remedy collection.

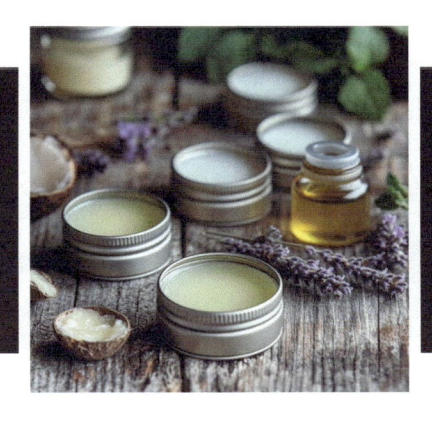

Ingredients:

- Coconut Oil: 1/2 cup (acts as a base and moisturizer)
- Beeswax: 2 tablespoons (helps solidify the salve)
- Lemon Eucalyptus Oil: 10 drops (known to repel mosquitoes)
- Lavender Oil: 8 drops (soothes skin and repels insects)
- Peppermint Oil: 6 drops (a powerful insect deterrent)
- Tea Tree Oil: 4 drops (natural repellent)

Instructions:

1. Melt the beeswax and coconut oil together in a double boiler.
2. Once melted, remove from heat and add the essential oils.
3. Stir well to combine, then pour the mixture into small tins or jars.
4. Allow to cool and solidify before use.
- Apply a small amount of salve directly to exposed skin and rub in gently. Reapply as needed, especially after sweating or swimming, to ensure continued protection from mosquitoes. Store in a cool, dry place.

Plantain & Coconut Itch Relief Balm

This simple yet effective anti-itch band aid uses plantain, a widely recognized herb for soothing skin irritations. The natural properties of plantain help relieve itching, reduce inflammation, and promote healing, making it a perfect remedy for minor rashes, insect bites, and other skin irritations.

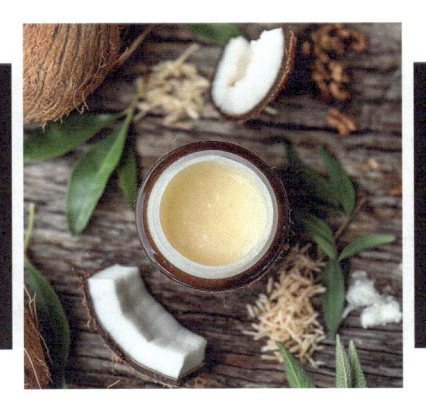

Ingredients:

- Fresh Plantain Leaves (4-6 leaves): Known for their anti-inflammatory and healing properties.
- Coconut Oil (1 tablespoon): Moisturizes and supports healing.
- Tea Tree Oil (3-4 drops): Acts as an antiseptic and antifungal.
- Beeswax (1 tablespoon): Helps to thicken the ointment for easy application.

Instructions:

1. Gather fresh plantain leaves, wash them well, and crush or chop them to release the juices.
2. In a pot, gently melt beeswax and coconut oil together.
3. Once the mixture is melted, add the plantain leaves and let them steep for about 10 minutes, stirring occasionally.
4. After removing from heat, add tea tree oil and mix thoroughly.
5. Pour into small containers, or if using immediately, apply the mixture directly onto the skin and cover with a clean cloth or bandage.
- Apply to the affected skin areas as needed to relieve itching. Reapply after a few hours if needed, especially if the bandage becomes wet. Store in a cool, dry place and use within a few weeks for the best results.

Antiseptic Ointment

This Antiseptic Ointment is designed to help cleanse and protect minor cuts, scrapes, and insect bites. It uses powerful herbs known for their antimicrobial and soothing properties, making it a staple in natural first-aid care.

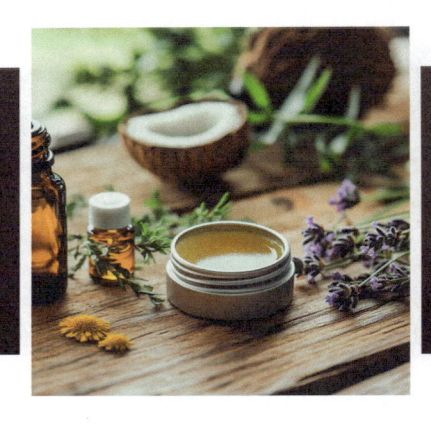

Ingredients:

- Tea Tree Oil: A natural antiseptic, helps kill bacteria and reduce inflammation.
- Lavender Oil: Known for its calming and antibacterial effects, soothes and aids skin recovery.
- Beeswax: Creates a protective barrier on the skin while locking in moisture.
- Coconut Oil: Moisturizes and has mild antimicrobial properties to support wound care.
- Calendula Oil: Known for its skin-soothing and healing properties, helps reduce redness and irritation.

Instructions:

1. In a double boiler, melt 2 tablespoons of beeswax with 1/4 cup of coconut oil.
2. Remove from heat and stir in 10 drops each of tea tree and lavender oils, and 1 tablespoon of calendula oil.
3. Pour the mixture into a clean, small tin or jar and allow it to cool and solidify.
- Apply a thin layer of balm directly to clean skin on cuts, scrapes, or bug bites as needed. Reapply 1-2 times daily to keep the area moisturized and protected.

Herbal Wound Care Elixir

This natural antiseptic solution is inspired by the properties of betadine but uses gentle, plant-based ingredients. It can be used for minor cuts, scrapes, and wounds to help prevent infection and promote healing.

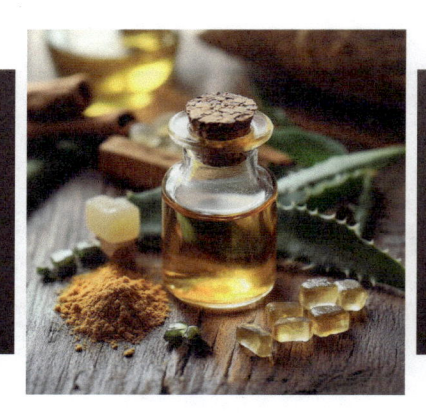

Ingredients:

- Goldenseal Powder: Known for its antimicrobial and antiseptic qualities, helps disinfect the wound area.
- Myrrh Resin: An ancient remedy with antiseptic and anti-inflammatory properties, supporting wound cleansing.
- Tea Tree Oil: Offers natural antibacterial and antifungal benefits, effective against various pathogens.
- Aloe Vera Gel: Soothes the skin, promotes healing, and provides moisture to aid the skin's recovery.

Instructions:

1. In a small sterilized bottle, combine 1 tablespoon of aloe vera gel with 1/4 teaspoon of goldenseal powder.
2. Add 5 drops of tea tree oil and a pinch of myrrh resin powder, then shake the bottle to mix thoroughly.
3. Let the mixture sit for a few hours to allow the ingredients to blend.
- Cleanse the wound, then apply a few drops of the mixture directly to the area with a sterile cotton swab. Repeat once or twice daily until the wound begins to heal.

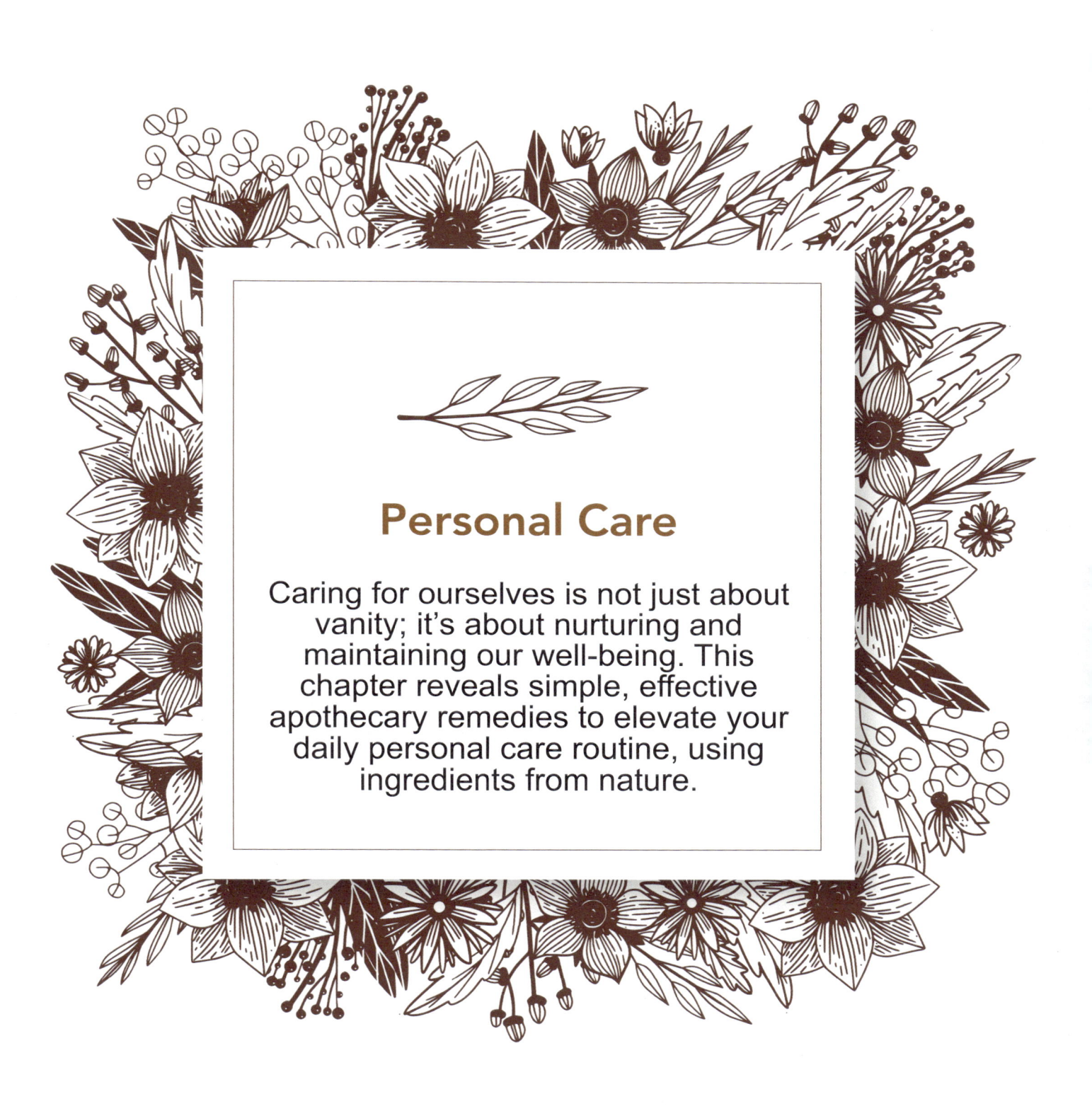

Personal Care

Caring for ourselves is not just about vanity; it's about nurturing and maintaining our well-being. This chapter reveals simple, effective apothecary remedies to elevate your daily personal care routine, using ingredients from nature.

Herbal Hair Growth Tonic

Rosemary is a popular herb known for its ability to stimulate hair growth by improving circulation to the scalp and promoting stronger hair follicles. This Herbal Hair Growth Tonic can be easily made at home to support scalp health and encourage hair growth.

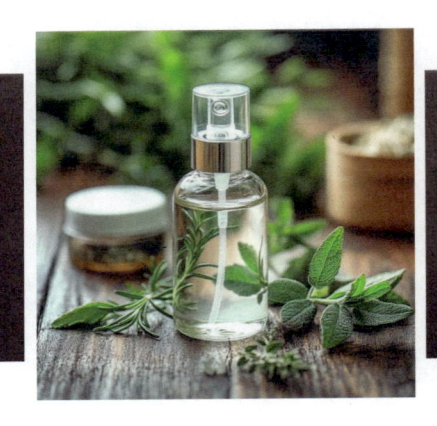

Ingredients:

- Rosemary Essential Oil (10-15 drops): Known for stimulating hair growth and improving circulation to the scalp.
- Peppermint Essential Oil (5-10 drops): Encourages blood flow to the scalp, which may support healthy hair growth.
- Witch Hazel (2 tablespoons): Acts as a natural astringent and helps the oils mix with water.
- Distilled Water (1 cup): Acts as a base for the spray.
- Aloe Vera Gel (optional, 1-2 tablespoons): Soothes and hydrates the scalp.

Instructions:

1. In a small spray bottle, combine 1 cup of distilled water and 2 tablespoons of witch hazel.
2. Add 10-15 drops of rosemary essential oil and 5-10 drops of peppermint essential oil to the mixture.
3. If using, add 1-2 tablespoons of aloe vera gel for added scalp hydration.
4. Shake the bottle well to mix the ingredients.
- Spray the mixture onto your scalp, especially targeting areas where hair growth is desired. Massage gently to improve absorption. Leave it in for at least 30 minutes, or overnight, and then wash as usual. For best results, use 2-3 times a week.

Age Spot Rejuvenation Balm

Arnica is well-known for its ability to improve skin appearance by reducing inflammation and promoting healing. This salve can be used to help fade age spots, as it encourages skin regeneration and enhances circulation, which may support the lightening of hyperpigmented spots over time.

Ingredients:

- Arnica Oil (2 tablespoons): Known for its anti-inflammatory and skin-healing properties.
- Coconut Oil (2 tablespoons): Moisturizes and softens the skin while allowing better absorption of the active ingredients.
- Beeswax (1 tablespoon): Helps to solidify the salve and acts as a natural barrier to protect the skin.
- Lavender Essential Oil (5 drops): Adds a soothing, healing element that promotes skin regeneration.

Instructions:

1. In a double boiler, gently heat the coconut oil and beeswax until melted.
2. Add the arnica oil or infused oil and stir to combine.
3. Remove from heat and add the lavender essential oil.
4. Pour the mixture into a small jar or tin and let it cool completely to solidify.
5. Store in a cool, dark place to preserve the potency of the oils.
- Apply a small amount of the salve to age spots once or twice a day. Gently massage into the skin until absorbed. Consistency is key, so use regularly for the best results. If irritation occurs, discontinue use and consult a healthcare provider.

Herbal Fresh Mint Toothpaste

This herbal toothpaste combines natural ingredients known for their ability to clean teeth, reduce inflammation, and support oral health. It's free from synthetic chemicals and focuses on using natural antibacterial and anti-inflammatory properties.

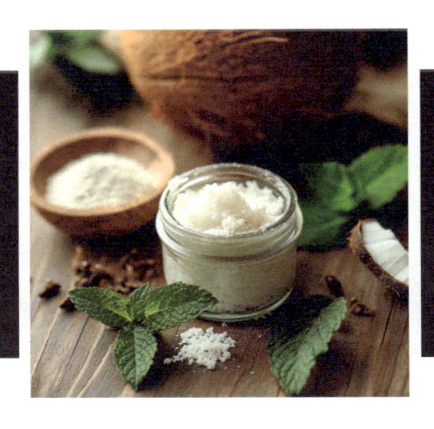

Ingredients:

- Coconut Oil (2 tablespoons): Moisturizes and helps fight bacteria due to its natural antimicrobial properties.
- Peppermint Essential Oil (5 drops): Provides a fresh, minty taste and helps with gum health and breath.
- Neem Powder (1 tablespoon): Known for its antibacterial properties that help maintain oral hygiene.
- Clove Powder (1 teaspoon): Offers antimicrobial effects and can soothe gum irritation.
- Baking Soda (2 tablespoons): Acts as a gentle abrasive that helps clean teeth and remove plaque.

Instructions:

1. In a small bowl, mix the baking soda, coconut oil, neem powder, and clove powder.
2. Add peppermint essential oil and stir well to form a paste-like consistency.
3. Store in a small glass jar with a tight-fitting lid.
- Apply a small amount of the toothpaste onto your toothbrush and brush as usual. Use morning and night for optimal oral health. This natural toothpaste helps clean teeth, freshen breath, and support gum health without harsh chemicals. If irritation occurs, discontinue use.

Herbal Gum Care Mouthwash

This natural mouthwash helps support gum health and strengthen the tissues of the mouth using ingredients known for their antibacterial, anti-inflammatory, and soothing properties.

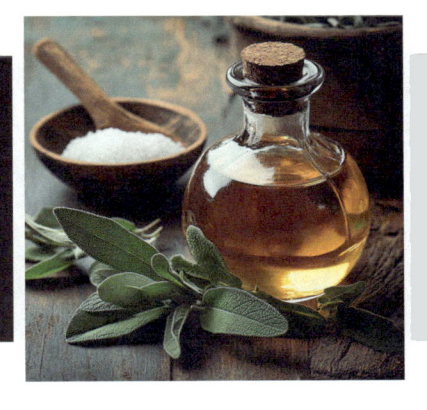

Ingredients:

- Sage Leaves (1 tablespoon): Known for its ability to reduce gum inflammation and fight oral bacteria.
- Peppermint Essential Oil (5 drops): Provides a fresh minty taste while helping to improve gum health and reduce bad breath.
- Apple Cider Vinegar (1 tablespoon): A natural cleanser that balances the pH of the mouth and supports gum health.
- Water (1 cup): Used as the base for the mouthwash.
- Salt (1 teaspoon): Helps reduce inflammation and supports oral health by killing bacteria.

Instructions:

1. Boil the water and steep the sage leaves in it for about 10 minutes.
2. Remove from heat and strain out the sage leaves.
3. Add the salt, apple cider vinegar, and peppermint essential oil to the cooled sage infusion.
4. Stir well to combine.
5. Store the mouthwash in a clean, airtight glass bottle.
- Swish 1–2 tablespoons of the mouthwash in your mouth for 30 seconds, focusing on the gums. Spit it out and rinse with clean water. Use once or twice daily, ideally after meals, for strengthening gums and maintaining fresh breath. If any irritation occurs, discontinue use.

Natural Youth Elixir

This natural remedy focuses on promoting youthful, plump skin by stimulating collagen production, tightening and hydrating the skin. It combines ingredients known for their skin rejuvenating properties to give a natural boost to your appearance, similar to the effects of botox but without the harsh chemicals or injections.

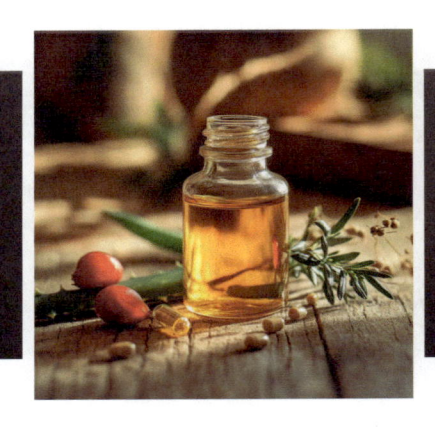

Ingredients:

- Rosehip Oil (1 tablespoon): Rich in essential fatty acids and antioxidants, rosehip oil helps improve skin elasticity and reduces wrinkles.
- Aloe Vera Gel (2 tablespoons): Known for its soothing and hydrating properties, aloe vera helps tighten skin and promotes healing.
- Jojoba Oil (1 teaspoon): Moisturizes the skin deeply and helps to reduce the appearance of fine lines.
- Vitamin E Oil (1 teaspoon): A powerful antioxidant that promotes collagen production and protects the skin from free radicals.
- Frankincense Essential Oil (2-3 drops): Known for its ability to regenerate skin cells and tighten the skin.

Instructions:

1. In a small bowl, combine the rosehip oil, aloe vera gel, and jojoba oil.
2. Add the vitamin E oil and frankincense essential oil, stirring well to blend all ingredients together.
3. Transfer the mixture to a small glass jar or bottle with an airtight lid.
- Apply a small amount of the mixture to clean, dry skin. Massage gently into areas that need tightening, such as around the eyes, mouth, and forehead. Use daily, preferably at night, to allow the oils to work overnight. After consistent use for a few weeks, you'll begin to notice smoother, firmer skin. Avoid using on broken or irritated skin.

Glow & Balance Face Elixir

This Glow & Balance Face Elixir blend is designed to nourish and rejuvenate the skin. It combines a variety of oils with unique properties to hydrate, balance, and heal the skin, making it perfect for daily use as part of your skincare routine.

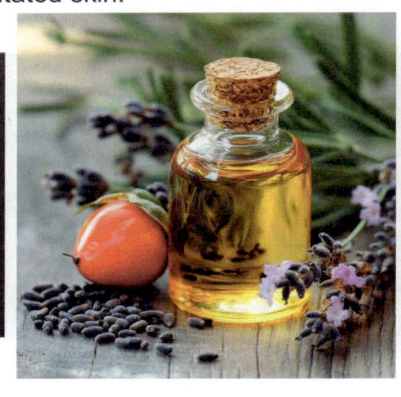

Ingredients:

- Jojoba Oil (2 tablespoons): A lightweight oil that closely resembles the skin's natural sebum, helping to balance oil production and hydrate the skin without clogging pores.
- Rosehip Oil (1 tablespoon): Rich in vitamin C and essential fatty acids, it helps to reduce the appearance of scars, fine lines, and promotes skin regeneration.
- Lavender Essential Oil (3-4 drops): Known for its calming properties, it soothes irritated skin, reduces redness, and promotes healing.
- Geranium Essential Oil (2-3 drops): Balances oil production, tightens the skin, and improves elasticity.
- Vitamin E Oil (1 teaspoon): An antioxidant that helps to repair skin damage, reduce fine lines, and improve skin texture.

Instructions:

1. In a small glass bottle, combine the jojoba oil, rosehip oil, and vitamin E oil.
2. Add the lavender and geranium essential oils to the bottle and shake well to mix.
3. Ensure the bottle is tightly sealed and store in a cool, dark place for optimal preservation.
- Apply a few drops of the oil to your fingertips and gently massage it into your face in upward motions, ideally after cleansing. Use this oil in the evening before bedtime for hydration and skin rejuvenation. You can also use it in the morning if your skin feels dry or needs extra moisture. This blend is great for all skin types, including sensitive skin.

Herbal Breeze Natural Deodorant

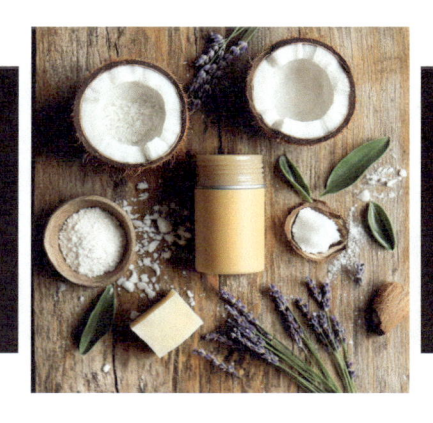

This Herbal Breeze Natural Deodorant is made with simple, skin-friendly ingredients that absorb moisture and neutralize odor, while being free from harsh chemicals. It's a great alternative to store-bought deodorants, offering long-lasting freshness and skin benefits.

Ingredients:

- Coconut Oil (3 tablespoons): Contains natural antibacterial properties, helping to combat odor-causing bacteria.
- Arrowroot Powder (2 tablespoons): Helps absorb moisture, keeping your skin dry without irritation.
- Beeswax (1 tablespoon): Provides structure to the stick and ensures it remains solid.
- Lavender Essential Oil (10 drops): Offers a fresh, calming scent, while providing soothing properties.
- Tea Tree Essential Oil (5 drops): helps fight the bacteria responsible for body odor.
- Baking Soda (2 tablespoons): Neutralizes odor and absorbs moisture.

Instructions:

1. In a double boiler, melt the beeswax and coconut oil together until fully combined.
2. Add the baking soda and arrowroot powder to the mixture, stirring to combine thoroughly.
3. Remove from heat and add the essential oils, mixing well.
4. Pour the mixture into an empty deodorant stick container and allow it to cool and harden for a few hours.
- Apply a thin layer to clean, dry underarms daily. This deodorant is gentle on the skin and works to keep you fresh without the use of harmful chemicals or synthetic fragrances. If you experience any irritation, discontinue use and adjust the formula as needed.

Herbal Sun Protect Lotion

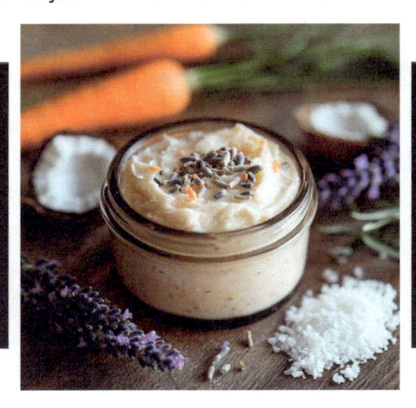

A homemade herbal sunscreen is a great way to protect your skin from the sun's harmful rays while nourishing and moisturizing. With natural ingredients, this recipe combines plant oils and zinc oxide to create a safe and effective alternative to chemical sunscreens.

Ingredients:

- Zinc Oxide (2 tablespoons): Provides physical sun protection by reflecting UV rays away from the skin.
- Coconut Oil (4 tablespoons): Naturally moisturizing and offers mild sun protection.
- Shea Butter (3 tablespoons): Hydrates and protects the skin, with mild SPF properties.
- Carrot Seed Oil (1 tablespoon): Contains antioxidants and natural SPF to enhance sun protection.
- Jojoba Oil (2 tablespoons): Moisturizes and supports healthy skin while balancing oil production.
- Lavender Essential Oil (5 drops): Calms and heals skin while adding a fresh scent.

Instructions:

1. In a double boiler, melt coconut oil and shea butter together.
2. Once melted, add jojoba oil and carrot seed oil to the mixture.
3. Slowly stir in zinc oxide, mixing thoroughly to avoid clumping.
4. Add the lavender essential oil and blend well.
5. Pour into a container and allow to cool and solidify.
- Apply liberally to exposed skin 15 minutes before sun exposure. Reapply every 2 hours, or after swimming, for continued protection.
-

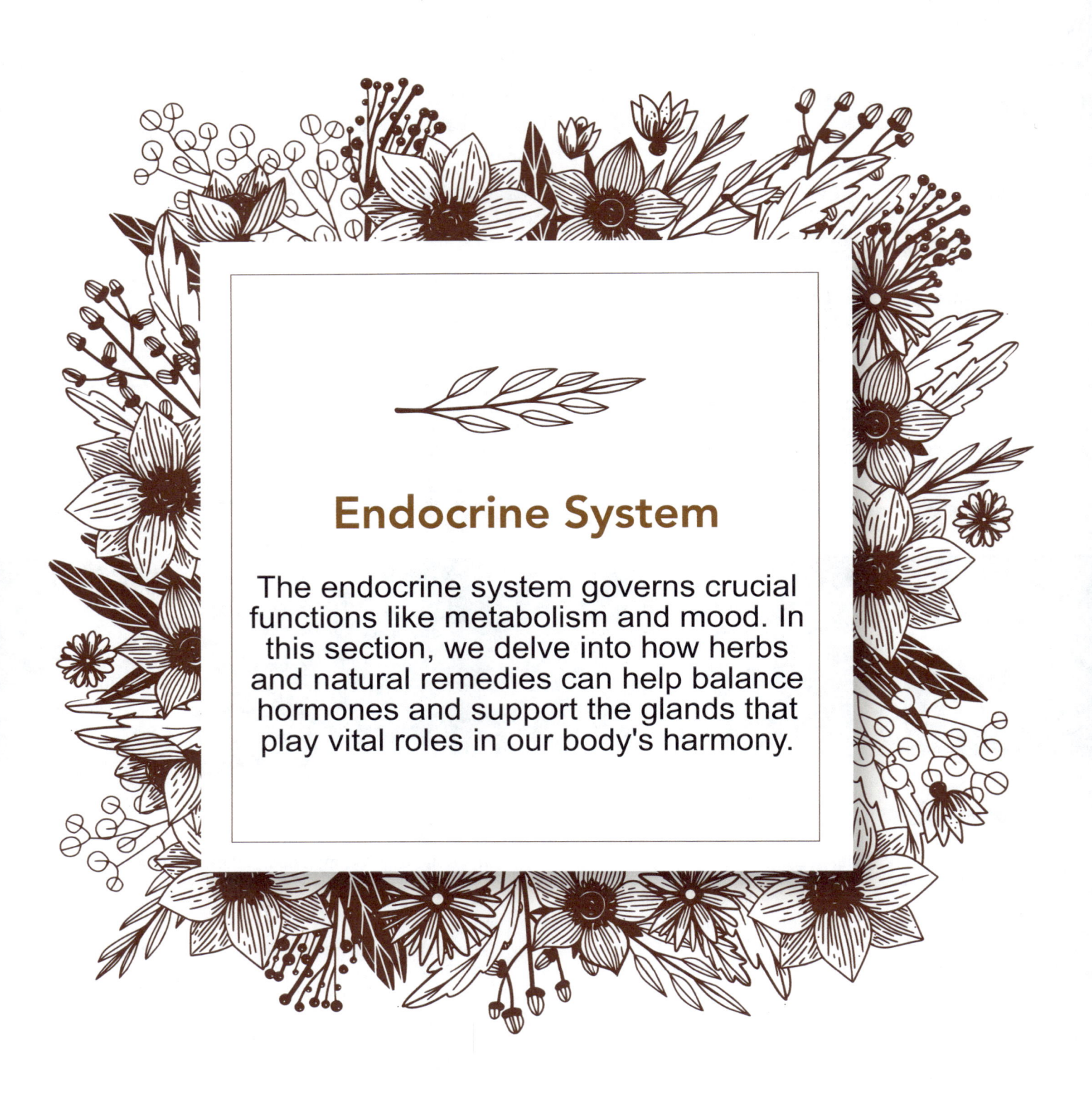

Endocrine System

The endocrine system governs crucial functions like metabolism and mood. In this section, we delve into how herbs and natural remedies can help balance hormones and support the glands that play vital roles in our body's harmony.

Nature's PCOS Aid

This herbal blend is crafted to help support hormonal balance, reduce inflammation, and promote overall wellness for individuals with Polycystic Ovary Syndrome (PCOS). Key herbs included have been traditionally used to support reproductive health and balance hormones naturally.

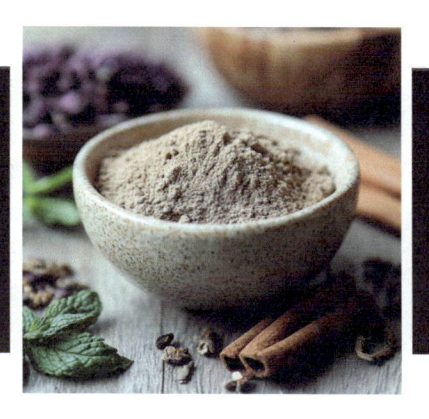

Ingredients:

- Chasteberry (Vitex) Powder (1 tsp): Known to support hormone regulation, especially for balancing progesterone and estrogen levels.
- Spearmint Leaves (1 tsp, dried): May help reduce androgen levels, which is beneficial for PCOS symptoms like unwanted hair growth.
- Licorice Root Powder (1/2 tsp): Contains anti-inflammatory compounds and may support hormone balance.
- Maca Root Powder (1/2 tsp): An adaptogen known for its ability to support endocrine health and reduce symptoms associated with hormonal imbalance.
- Cinnamon Powder (1/2 tsp): Can help with blood sugar regulation, a common concern for individuals with PCOS.

Instructions:

1. Mix all ingredients thoroughly in a small bowl.
2. Store the blend in an airtight container.

- Add 1 teaspoon of the blend to warm water, a smoothie, or herbal tea once daily. For best results, take consistently over several weeks and observe any changes.
- Keep the blend in a cool, dry place for up to six months.

Pancreas Support Spiced Milk

This blend combines warming spices traditionally used to promote digestive and metabolic health, aimed at supporting pancreas function. Turmeric, ginger, cinnamon, and cardamom are featured for their reputed anti-inflammatory and antioxidant properties, making this a calming, nourishing drink.

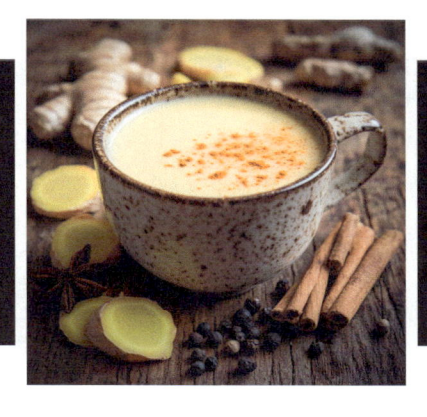

Ingredients:

- Turmeric (1/2 tsp): Contains curcumin, which may reduce inflammation and support healthy blood sugar.
- Ginger (1/4 tsp, powdered or fresh): Known for digestive benefits, ginger can soothe and balance.
- Cinnamon (1/4 tsp): Thought to support blood sugar levels and has warming effects.
- Black Pepper (a pinch): Enhances curcumin absorption from turmeric.
- Cardamom (a pinch): Eases digestion and balances the flavors.
- Milk (1 cup, warm): Acts as a calming carrier for the spices.

Instructions:

1. In a saucepan, combine all spices with the milk.
2. Heat on low, stirring, until it simmers, allowing flavors to infuse for 2–3 minutes.
3. Pour into a cup to cool slightly before drinking.

- Enjoy this drink once daily, especially in the evening. Adjust spices as desired.
- Prepare fresh each time for best effects and flavor.

Blood Sugar Balance Tea

This blend combines the blood sugar-balancing properties of bitter melon and the antioxidant benefits of green tea, traditionally used to support stable energy levels and metabolic health. Bitter melon contains compounds that may mimic insulin's effects, while green tea provides gentle stimulation and a high dose of antioxidants.

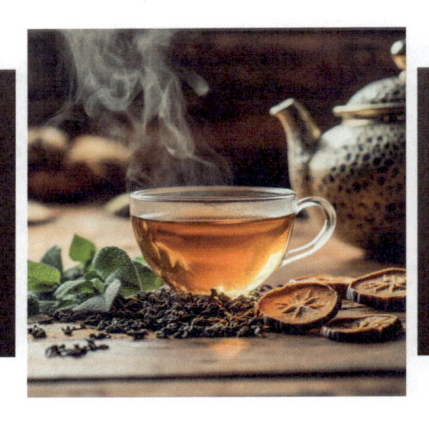

Ingredients:

- Dried Bitter Melon (1 tbsp, chopped): Contains polypeptide-p and charantin, which may help regulate blood sugar.
- Green Tea Leaves (1 tsp): Rich in catechins, known for their anti-inflammatory and blood sugar-regulating effects.
- Hot Water (1 cup): To infuse and extract the active compounds.

Instructions:

1. Add dried bitter melon and green tea leaves to a teapot or infuser.
2. Pour hot water over the mixture, letting it steep for 5–10 minutes.
3. Strain into a cup and let cool slightly before drinking.

- Drink this blend up to twice daily, preferably between meals, to support balanced blood sugar levels.

Rhodiola Stress Relief Capsules

Rhodiola (Rhodiola rosea) is an adaptogenic herb known for its ability to help the body cope with stress, balance cortisol levels, and increase energy. This herb supports overall adrenal function and can help reduce the negative effects of chronic stress on the body.

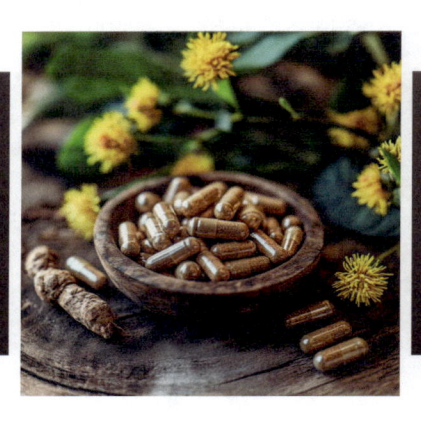

Ingredients:

- Rhodiola Root Powder (1–2 teaspoons): Known for its ability to regulate cortisol and improve resilience to stress.
- Empty Gelatin or Vegetable Capsules (size 00 or 000): To encapsulate the herb for easy consumption.

Instructions:

1. Fill the capsules with 1–2 teaspoons of dried Rhodiola root powder.
2. Seal the capsules tightly.
3. Store in a cool, dry place, away from direct sunlight.

- Take 1 capsule daily to support cortisol balance. For acute stress or fatigue, you can increase the dosage to 2–3 capsules per day, but do so gradually. It's best to start with a smaller dose and monitor how your body responds. Rhodiola is generally well-tolerated, but if you have any existing conditions or are on medication, consult a healthcare provider before starting this remedy.
- Keep in a dry, dark place, and consume within 6–12 months for optimal freshness.

Pancreas Health Herbal Blend

This herbal blend includes plants traditionally used to support pancreatic health and regulate blood sugar levels. Combining the benefits of bitter melon, turmeric, and fenugreek, this remedy may assist with maintaining balanced blood sugar and improving overall pancreatic function.

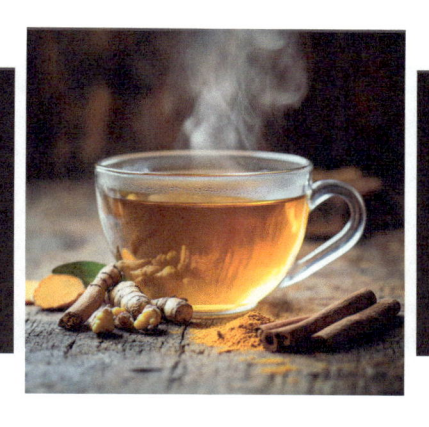

Ingredients:

- Bitter Melon: Known for its ability to help regulate blood sugar levels and support pancreatic function.
- Turmeric Root: Contains compounds that help reduce inflammation and support overall metabolic function.
- Fenugreek Seeds: Helps maintain balanced blood sugar levels and supports the pancreas.
- Cinnamon Bark: Regulates blood sugar and improves insulin sensitivity.

Instructions:

1. Add 1 tablespoon of the dried herbs to 2 cups of boiling water.
2. Let the mixture steep for 15–20 minutes.
3. Strain out the herbs and pour the liquid into a cup.

- Drink 1–2 cups daily, preferably after meals, to support pancreatic health and blood sugar balance. For best results, continue for several weeks.
- Keep dried herbs in an airtight container in a cool, dry place for optimal potency.
- For those with existing health conditions or medications, consult a healthcare provider before use.

Hormonal Harmony Tea

This herbal elixir is designed to support hormonal balance, particularly for those experiencing PMS, menopause symptoms, or hormonal imbalances. It combines herbs traditionally used for their ability to regulate hormone levels and improve overall wellness.

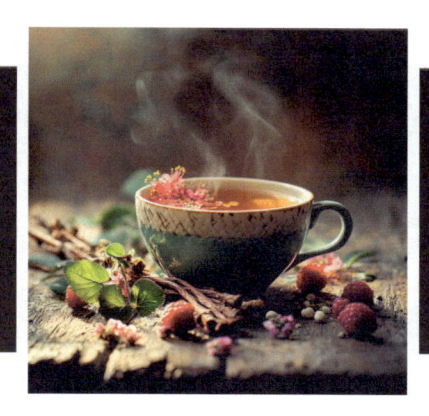

Ingredients:

- Chaste Tree Berry: Supports progesterone production and helps balance hormones, especially beneficial for women with irregular cycles or PMS.
- Dong Quai Root: Often used to support female reproductive health and relieve menstrual discomfort.
- Licorice Root: Supports adrenal health and helps balance cortisol levels, which can improve overall hormonal harmony.
- Red Clover: Rich in isoflavones, which may help balance estrogen levels and support menopause symptoms.
- Raspberry Leaf: Known for its ability to tone the uterus and regulate menstrual cycles.

Instructions:

1. Combine 1 tablespoon of each dried herb in a glass jar.
2. Pour 2 cups of hot water over the herbs and cover with a lid.
3. Let steep for 15–20 minutes.
4. Strain and store the liquid in a glass bottle.

- Drink 1 cup daily, especially during the luteal phase of the menstrual cycle or when experiencing hormonal fluctuations. For best results, continue for at least a month.
- Keep refrigerated for up to a week, or store in a cool, dark place for up to 3 days.

Gut Soother Infusion

Bugleweed (Lycopus virginicus) has traditionally been used to help manage thyroid imbalances, particularly in cases of hyperthyroidism. This herb is known for its ability to support thyroid health by potentially inhibiting excess thyroid hormone production, making it useful for conditions like Graves' disease and hyperthyroidism.

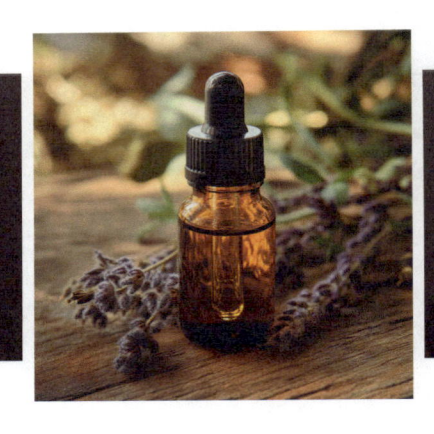

Ingredients:

- Bugleweed (Lycopus virginicus) (1 cup dried herb): Known for its ability to balance thyroid function by inhibiting excessive hormone production.
- Vegetable Glycerin (2 cups): A gentle, alcohol-free extraction medium that helps preserve the medicinal properties of the herb.

Instructions:

1. Fill a clean glass jar halfway with dried bugleweed leaves.
2. Pour vegetable glycerin over the herb, covering it completely. Leave about an inch of space at the top of the jar.
3. Seal the jar tightly and shake well.
4. Store the jar in a cool, dark place for 4–6 weeks. Shake the jar daily to mix the herb with the glycerin. After 4–6 weeks, strain the liquid through a fine mesh strainer or cheesecloth into a clean bottle.
- Take 1–2 droppers of the glycerite up to three times daily to support thyroid balance. Begin with a smaller dose and increase gradually as needed.

Bladderwrack Tincture for Thyroid Support

Bladderwrack (Fucus vesiculosus) is a seaweed rich in iodine, an essential mineral for thyroid function. This tincture is commonly used to support underactive thyroid conditions, as iodine plays a key role in thyroid hormone production.

Ingredients:

- Dried Bladderwrack (1 cup): High in iodine, which supports thyroid function, especially beneficial for hypothyroid concerns.
- Vegetable Glycerin (1 cup): Acts as the base for the tincture, creating a gentle, alcohol-free extract.
- Water (1 cup): Dilutes the glycerin, aiding in the extraction process.

Instructions:

1. Combine equal parts vegetable glycerin and water to form a 50/50 mixture.
2. Place dried bladderwrack in a clean glass jar and pour the glycerin-water mixture over it, fully covering the herb.
3. Seal the jar tightly, shake well, and store it in a cool, dark place for 4–6 weeks, shaking it daily.
4. After extraction, strain the glycerite through cheesecloth or a fine strainer into a clean bottle.
- Take 10–15 drops up to twice daily, diluted in water, to support thyroid function. Start with a low dose and observe how you feel, adjusting as needed. Consult a healthcare provider before use, especially if you have thyroid conditions or sensitivities.

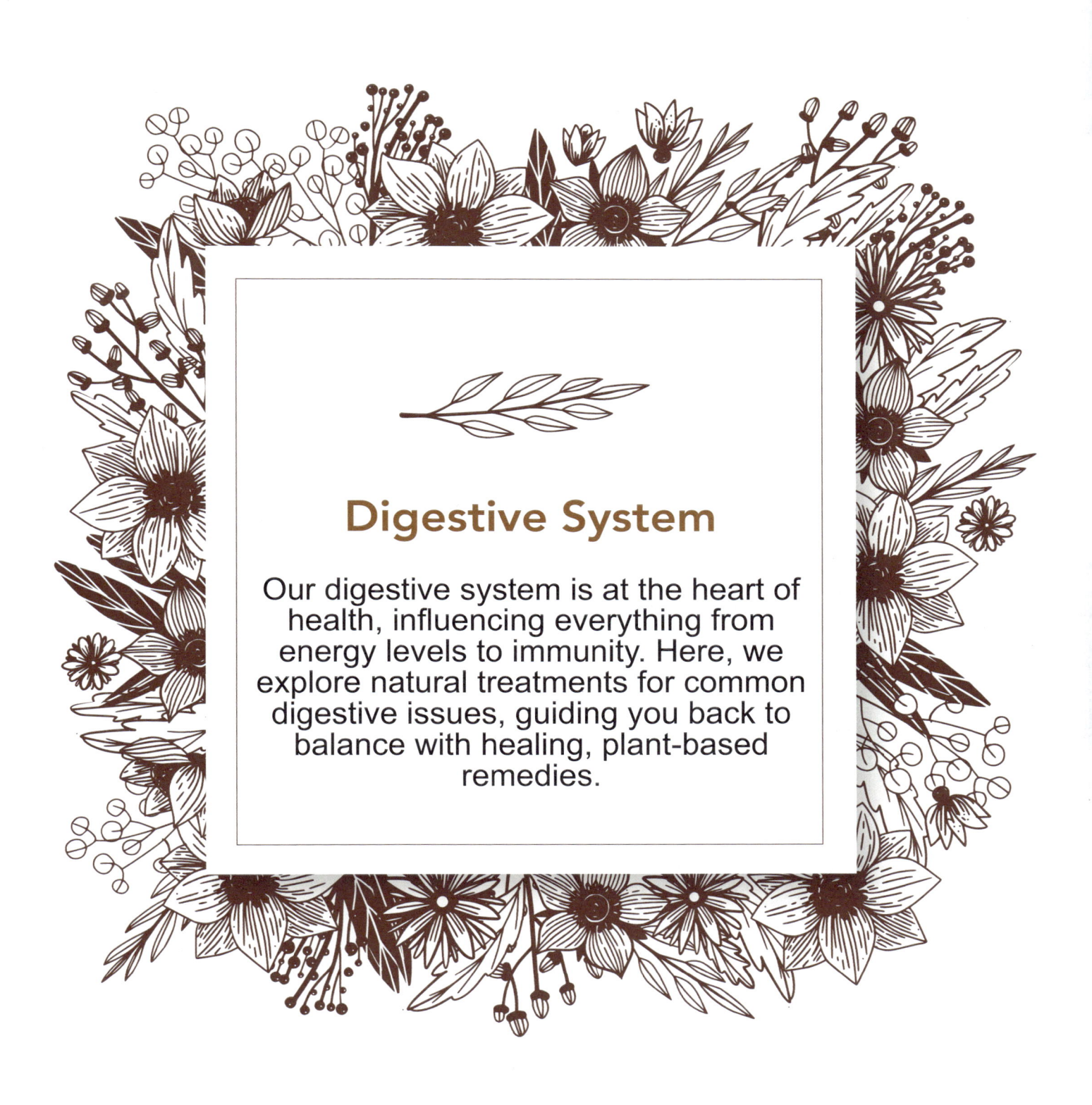

Digestive System

Our digestive system is at the heart of health, influencing everything from energy levels to immunity. Here, we explore natural treatments for common digestive issues, guiding you back to balance with healing, plant-based remedies.

Black Milk

Black Milk is an ancient herbal drink traditionally used for its cooling, detoxifying, and calming properties. It's especially popular for its potential to support digestion, improve skin health, and help balance bodily systems. Typically made from herbal ingredients, this beverage is rich in minerals and vitamins.

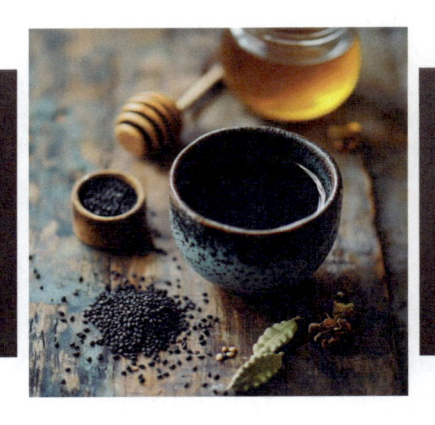

Ingredients:

- Black Sesame Seeds: High in calcium, magnesium, and healthy fats, they promote bone health, improve digestion, and benefit skin appearance.
- Cumin: Aids in digestion, detoxifies, and supports metabolic function.
- Cardamom: Soothes the digestive system, helps with circulation, and supports detoxification.
- Honey: Adds sweetness while providing antimicrobial and immune-boosting properties.
- Milk or Non-Dairy Alternative: Acts as a smooth base for the drink, aiding in digestion and providing a creamy texture.

Instructions:

1. Toast 1 tablespoon black sesame seeds until aromatic, then grind into a powder.
2. Heat 1 cup of milk or non-dairy alternative.
3. Add 1/4 teaspoon cumin and cardamom, along with 1 tablespoon ground sesame seeds.
4. Sweeten with honey and simmer for 5–10 minutes. Then strain and serve warm.
- Drink 1–2 times a day, especially in the evening, to help calm the digestive system, promote relaxation, and nourish the skin.
- Store leftovers in the refrigerator for up to 24 hours. Reheat gently before drinking.

Gut Soother Infusion

This soothing herbal infusion supports digestive health and helps relieve bloating, gas, and discomfort. The blend of peppermint, ginger, fennel, and licorice root is traditionally used to calm the stomach and promote healthy digestion.

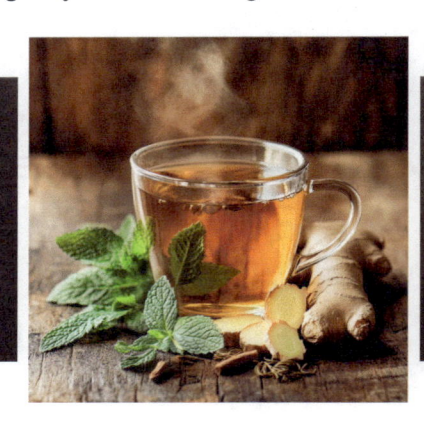

Ingredients:

- Peppermint Leaves (1 tablespoon): Helps relieve digestive discomfort and reduce bloating.
- Ginger Root (1 teaspoon, freshly grated): Soothes the stomach and supports digestion.
- Fennel Seeds (1 teaspoon): Eases gas and bloating, promoting smoother digestion.
- Licorice Root (1/2 teaspoon): Soothes the intestinal lining and promotes digestion.

Instructions:

1. Place all ingredients into a teapot or heatproof jar.
2. Pour 2 cups of boiling water over the herbs and cover.
3. Let steep for 10-15 minutes, then strain.

- Drink 1–2 cups daily after meals for digestive relief.
- This infusion can help ease discomfort and promote regular digestion. Keep any leftovers in the fridge for up to 24 hours.

Gut Detox Herbal Flush

This herbal flush combines potent anti-parasitic herbs traditionally used to cleanse the body of parasites. The blend of wormwood, black walnut hulls, and cloves has been passed down through generations to support digestive health and detoxification.

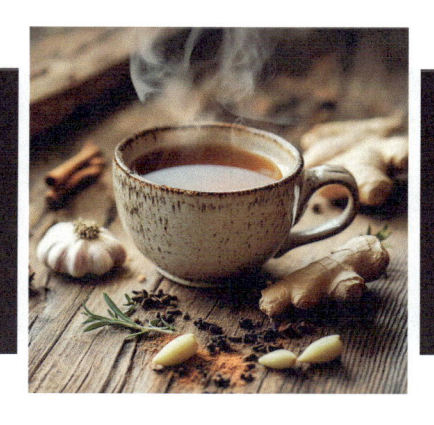

Ingredients:

- Wormwood (1 tablespoon): A powerful herb known to expel intestinal parasites and promote healthy digestion.
- Black Walnut Hulls (1 tablespoon): Contains juglone, which is believed to help eliminate parasites and support gut health.
- Clove Buds (1 teaspoon): Has natural compounds that help kill parasite eggs and promote digestive wellness.
- Ginger Root (1 teaspoon, freshly grated): Aids in digestion and enhances the body's ability to expel parasites.
- Garlic (2 cloves, crushed): Known for its antimicrobial properties, garlic can help eliminate harmful microorganisms in the digestive system.

Instructions:

1. Combine all herbs in a heatproof jar.
2. Pour 2 cups of boiling water over the herbs and let steep for 10-15 minutes.
3. Strain and drink 1 cup daily for 7-10 days to help flush out parasites.
- This Gut Detox Herbal Flush is a gentle way to support your body in ridding itself of unwanted invaders. However, always consult with a healthcare provider before starting any detox program.

Fermented Cabbage Elixir (Best Probiotic)

Fermented Cabbage Elixir is an excellent natural source of probiotics, beneficial for supporting gut health, digestion, and immunity. The fermentation process develops beneficial bacteria that help balance the gut microbiome.

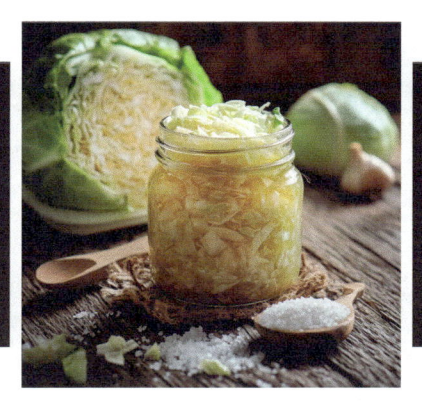

Ingredients:

- Cabbage (1 small head): Rich in fiber and nutrients that feed beneficial gut bacteria.
- Salt (1 tablespoon): Aids in the fermentation process and helps inhibit harmful bacteria.

Instructions:

1. Chop cabbage and add to a large bowl, sprinkling salt on top.
2. Massage the cabbage with hands until it releases liquid (about 10 minutes).
3. Pack the cabbage tightly into a jar, pressing down to submerge it in its own juices.
4. Cover the jar with a lid (loose) and let it ferment at room temperature for 3-5 days, checking for bubbling.
5. Once fermented, strain out the juice and store it in the fridge.
- Drink 1-2 ounces daily as a probiotic boost.

Natural Yarrow Bloat Extract

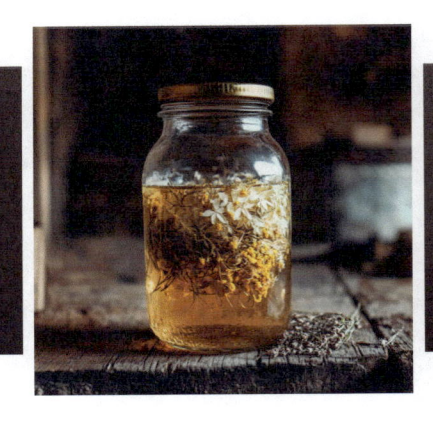

Yarrow extract is known for its anti-inflammatory and digestive-supporting properties, which can help alleviate bloating and ease digestive discomfort. This gentle herbal extract supports digestion by promoting bile flow and reducing gas.

Ingredients:

- Dried Yarrow (1 cup): Known for easing digestive discomfort and bloating.
- Apple Cider Vinegar (2 cups): Acts as a non-alcoholic solvent to draw out yarrow's beneficial compounds, while adding mild digestive support.

Instructions:

1. Place dried yarrow in a clean glass jar.
2. Pour apple cider vinegar over the yarrow until fully submerged, leaving space at the top.
3. Seal the jar tightly, shake, and store in a cool, dark place for 4-6 weeks, shaking gently every few days.
4. Strain the liquid into a clean bottle.

- Take 10–15 drops diluted in water before meals to help with bloating.
- Keep in a cool, dark place for up to a year.

Hemorrhoid Soothing Elixir

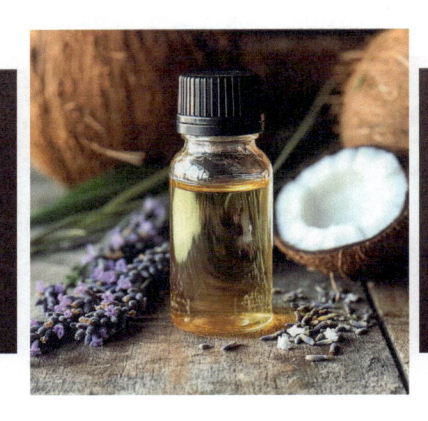

This soothing blend of oils is designed to reduce inflammation, relieve itching, and promote healing for hemorrhoids.

Ingredients:

- Witch Hazel Extract (2 tablespoons): Known for its anti-inflammatory properties, reduces swelling and soothes irritation.
- Coconut Oil (2 tablespoons): Moisturizes and has natural antibacterial properties.
- Chamomile Essential Oil (5 drops): Calms skin irritation and promotes healing.
- Lavender Essential Oil (5 drops): Helps reduce itching and discomfort.

Instructions:

1. In a small bowl, combine witch hazel extract and coconut oil.
2. Add chamomile and lavender essential oils, stirring well.
3. Pour the mixture into a clean glass bottle.

- Apply a small amount of oil to the affected area using a cotton pad, 1-2 times daily.
- Keep in a cool, dark place.

Soothing Digestive Kombucha

This homemade herbal kombucha combines probiotics with soothing herbs to support digestion, improve gut flora, and promote overall health.

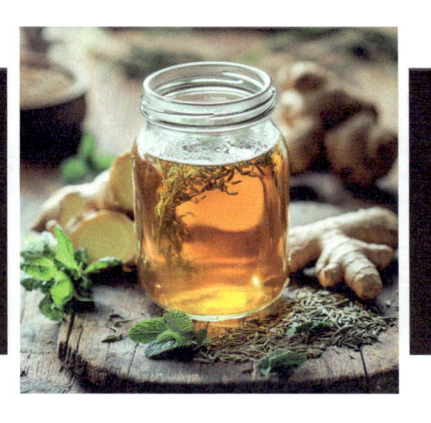

Ingredients:

- Green Tea (4 cups): Traditional tea base for kombucha, provides antioxidants and caffeine to fuel fermentation.
- Sugar (¼ cup): Feeds the fermentation process, broken down by bacteria and yeast.
- Scoby (1): The symbiotic culture of bacteria and yeast essential for fermentation.
- Ginger Root (1-inch piece): Supports digestion and adds a warming flavor.
- Peppermint (1 tablespoon, dried): Soothes the digestive tract.
- Fennel Seeds (1 teaspoon): Helps relieve bloating and supports gut health.

Instructions:

1. Brew the tea in hot water, add sugar, and let cool completely.
2. Pour the tea into a large jar, add the scoby, and cover with a cloth.
3. Let ferment for 7-10 days at room temperature, tasting for preferred tartness.
4. Remove scoby and add ginger, peppermint, and fennel for a second ferment.
5. Seal and ferment for an additional 1-3 days, then strain and refrigerate.
- Drink 4-8 ounces daily to support gut health.
- Store in the refrigerator and consume within two weeks.

4-Ingredient Digestive Elixir

This simple tonic aids digestion and soothes an upset stomach. The ingredients are carefully chosen for their digestive benefits and minimalism.

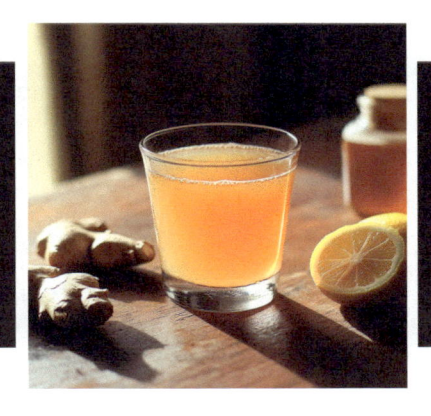

Ingredients:

- Apple Cider Vinegar (1 tbsp): Balances stomach pH and stimulates digestion.
- Ginger (1/2 tsp, grated): Reduces nausea and promotes stomach health.
- Lemon (juice of 1/2 lemon): Provides vitamin C and aids in digestion.
- Honey (1 tsp): Adds a touch of sweetness and soothes the digestive tract.

Instructions:

1. Mix all ingredients in a glass of warm water.
2. Stir well until honey dissolves.

- Sip slowly before or after meals to support digestion.
- Freshly prepare each time, as it's best consumed right after mixing.

Peaceful Night Infusion

A gentle, relaxing blend to soothe the mind and body, perfect for easing stress and promoting restful sleep.

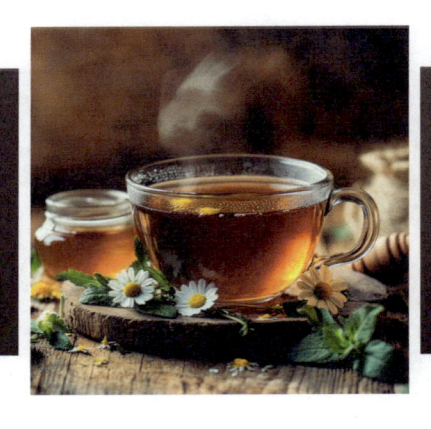

Ingredients:

- Chamomile (1 tbsp): Known for its calming effects and ability to support relaxation.
- Lemon Balm (1 tbsp): Helps reduce anxiety and stress, and supports a restful night's sleep.
- Honey (optional, 1 tsp): Adds natural sweetness and calming properties.
- Hot Water (1 cup)

Instructions:

- Add chamomile and lemon balm to a cup of hot water.
- Let steep for 5–10 minutes, then strain.
- Sip slowly in the evening to relax.
- Best consumed fresh.

Upset Stomach Comfort Syrup

This gentle, comforting syrup helps ease stomach discomfort, reduce nausea, and support digestion with a blend of soothing herbs.

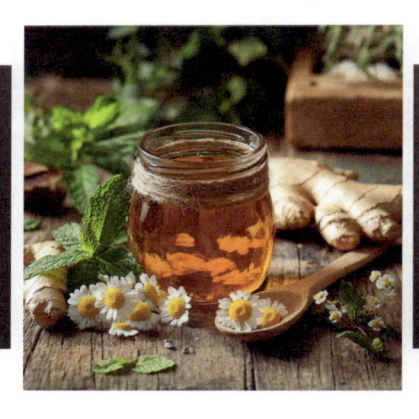

Ingredients:

- Ginger root (1 tbsp, grated): Known for its strong anti-nausea and digestion-supporting properties.
- Chamomile (1 tbsp): Calms the stomach and reduces tension.
- Peppermint (1 tsp): Eases digestion and reduces bloating.
- Honey (1 tbsp): Adds sweetness and has anti-inflammatory effects.
- Water (1 cup)

Instructions:

- Combine ginger, chamomile, and peppermint in water. Simmer for 10–15 minutes, then strain.
- Add honey to the warm mixture and stir until dissolved.
- Take 1–2 teaspoons as needed to soothe stomach discomfort.
- Store in the refrigerator for up to one week.

Lemon and Ginger Nausea Lollipops

These lollipops combine the soothing and anti-nausea properties of lemon and ginger into a sweet and convenient form, perfect for on-the-go relief.

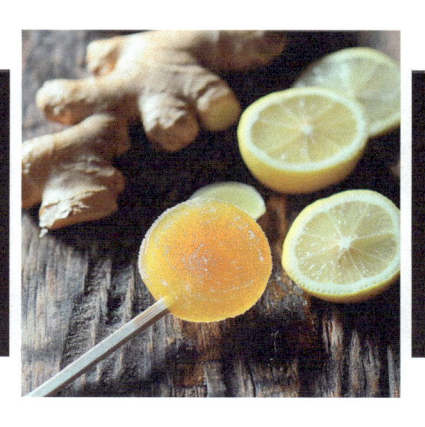

Ingredients:

- Fresh ginger (1 tbsp, grated)
- Lemon juice (2 tbsp)
- Honey (1/4 cup)
- Sugar (1 cup)
- Water (1/4 cup)
- Lollipop sticks or molds

Instructions:

1. Mix all ingredients in a saucepan.
2. Heat over medium heat, stirring occasionally until sugar dissolves and mixture reaches 300°F (hard candy stage).
3. Pour mixture into lollipop molds and insert sticks.
4. Let cool and harden completely.

- Sip on a lollipop whenever feeling nauseous.
- Store in an airtight container for up to 2 weeks.

Restorative Liver Tea

This soothing herbal tea is crafted to support liver function, detoxify the body, and promote overall health. The blend of liver-friendly herbs helps nurture and cleanse the liver while providing a calming, restorative experience.

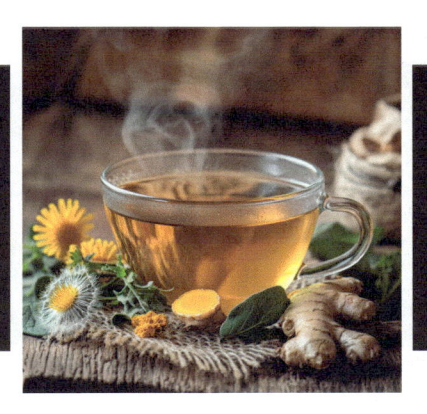

Ingredients:

- Dandelion root (1 tbsp): Known for its liver detoxification and diuretic properties.
- Milk thistle (1 tbsp): Supports liver health and regeneration of liver cells.
- Turmeric (1/2 tsp): Reduces inflammation and supports liver detox.
- Ginger (1 tsp, grated): Aids digestion and supports liver health.
- Lemon (juice of 1 lemon): Provides vitamin C and supports liver detoxification.
- Honey (1 tsp): A soothing sweetener with anti-inflammatory properties.

Instructions:

- Mix all ingredients in a glass of warm water.
- Stir well until honey dissolves.

- Sip slowly throughout the day, especially before or after meals, to support liver health.
- Freshly prepare each time, as it's best consumed right after mixing.

Fatty Liver Tincture

This tincture combines liver-supporting herbs that can help alleviate fatty liver symptoms, enhance liver function, and support detoxification. These ingredients are known to aid in reducing liver fat, inflammation, and promoting digestion.

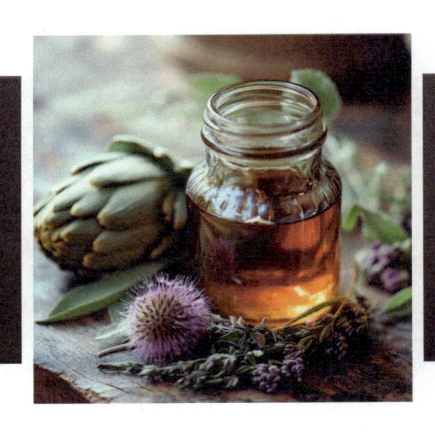

Ingredients:

- Milk Thistle Seeds (1 tablespoon): Contains silymarin, known to support liver cell regeneration and reduce inflammation.
- Dandelion Root (1 tablespoon, dried): Stimulates bile production to aid in liver detoxification and digestion.
- Artichoke Leaf (1 teaspoon): Known to support liver health and reduce fatty deposits in the liver.
- Apple Cider Vinegar (1 cup): Serves as a gentle solvent to extract the herbs' beneficial compounds.

Instructions:

1. Combine milk thistle seeds, dandelion root, and artichoke leaf in a clean jar.
2. Pour apple cider vinegar over the herbs, ensuring they are fully covered.
3. Seal the jar and store it in a cool, dark place for 2-3 weeks, shaking it daily.
4. After 2-3 weeks, strain and transfer the tincture to a clean bottle.
- Take 1-2 teaspoons daily to support liver health and aid digestion.
- Store in a cool, dark place. Use within 6 months.

Moringa Powder for Liver Detox

Moringa is a potent superfood that supports liver health by promoting detoxification and protecting against oxidative stress. This natural powder is packed with nutrients, antioxidants, and anti-inflammatory compounds that can help cleanse the liver and enhance overall liver function.

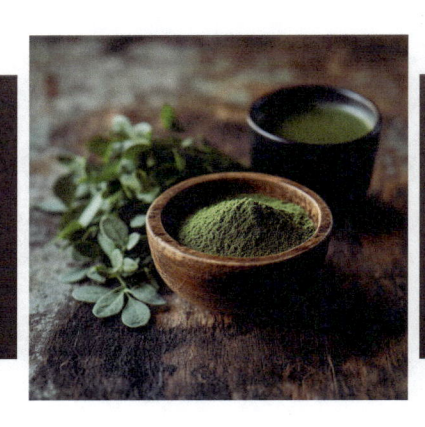

Ingredients:

- Moringa Powder (1-2 tsp): Known for its detoxifying properties and ability to support liver health.
- Water or Juice (1 cup): To help dissolve and ingest the powder.

Instructions:

1. Mix moringa powder with warm water or juice.
2. Stir well until completely dissolved.

- Drink once a day, preferably in the morning, to support liver detox and overall wellness.
- Store in a cool, dry place. Best used within 6 months.

Peppermint Ease for IBS

Peppermint oil has long been used to alleviate symptoms of irritable bowel syndrome (IBS), including bloating, cramping, and discomfort. Its menthol content helps to relax the muscles in the intestines, improving digestion and reducing pain.

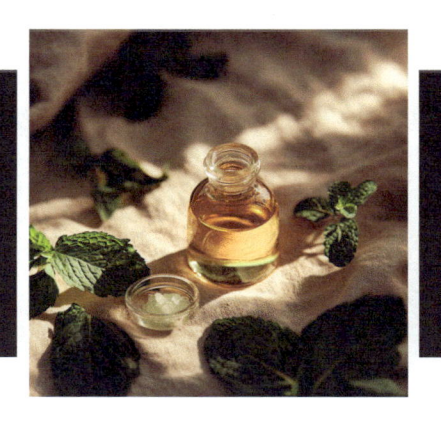

Ingredients:

- Peppermint Essential Oil (2-3 drops): Known for its ability to reduce IBS symptoms like bloating and cramping.
- Carrier Oil (like coconut or olive oil, 1 tsp): To dilute the essential oil and make it safe for topical use.

Instructions:

1. Mix the peppermint oil with a carrier oil.
2. Massage gently into the abdomen, focusing on the areas of discomfort.

- Apply 2-3 times daily to ease IBS symptoms or whenever needed for relief.
- Store in a cool, dry place, away from direct sunlight. Use within 6 months.
- Peppermint oil is a well-known remedy, but if you're new to essential oils or have any pre-existing conditions, consult with a healthcare provider before use.

Dandelion & Gentian Digestive Tonic

This digestive tonic combines the bitter properties of dandelion and gentian to stimulate the production of digestive juices, promoting healthy digestion and alleviating symptoms of indigestion, bloating, and discomfort.

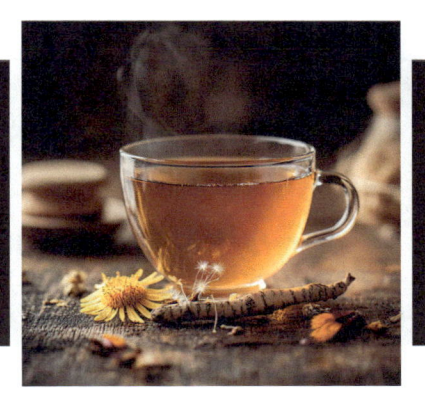

Ingredients:

- Dandelion Root (1 tablespoon): Known to support liver function and stimulate bile production, aiding digestion.
- Gentian Root (1 teaspoon): A bitter herb that enhances digestion by stimulating the secretion of digestive enzymes and bile.
- Honey (1 teaspoon): To balance the bitterness and add a soothing touch.
- Water (1 cup): For steeping the herbs.

Instructions:

1. Mix the dandelion and gentian root in a cup of hot water.
2. Let it steep for 10-15 minutes.
3. Strain the herbs, then add honey and stir until dissolved.

- Sip the tonic slowly before or after meals to aid digestion.
- Freshly prepare each time, as it's best consumed right after mixing.

Ginger & ACV for Bloating and Gas Relief

This soothing remedy combines ginger, a natural anti-inflammatory and digestive aid, with apple cider vinegar (ACV), known for its ability to promote digestion and balance stomach acids, helping to relieve bloating and gas.

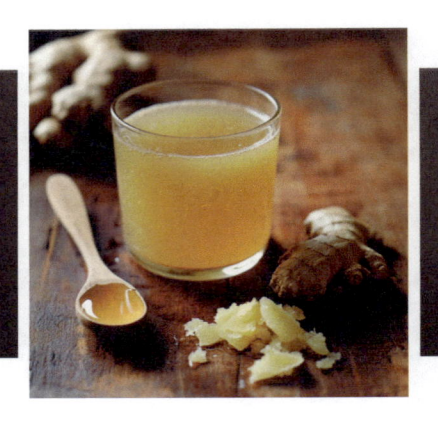

Ingredients:

- Fresh Ginger (1 teaspoon, grated): A natural anti-inflammatory that can reduce bloating and gas by promoting healthy digestion.
- Apple Cider Vinegar (1 tablespoon): Helps balance stomach acids, stimulates digestion, and can reduce bloating.
- Honey (1 teaspoon): To sweeten and soothe the stomach.
- Water (1 cup): For mixing and dilution.

Instructions:

1. Mix the ginger and ACV in a cup of warm water.
2. Add honey and stir until dissolved.

- Sip slowly before or after meals to reduce bloating and gas.
- Freshly prepare each time, as it's best consumed right after mixing.

Dandelion Lemonade for Gallbladder Health

This refreshing dandelion lemonade is a natural detoxifier, crafted with dandelion root, which is known to promote healthy liver and gallbladder function. The addition of lemon boosts the body's natural detoxification process and aids in digestion.

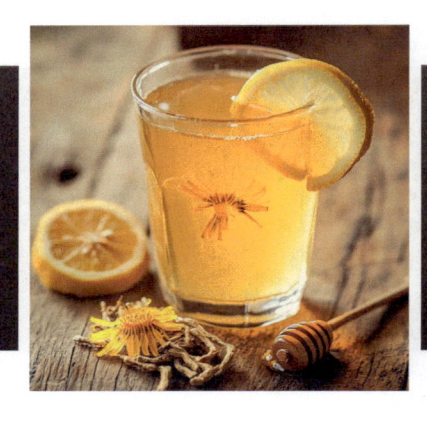

Ingredients:

- Dandelion Root (1 tablespoon, dried or fresh): Supports liver and gallbladder health by stimulating bile production, which helps in digestion and detoxification.
- Lemon Juice (juice of 1 lemon): Rich in vitamin C and antioxidants, aids in detoxification and supports liver function.
- Honey (1 teaspoon): For sweetness and to soothe the digestive tract.
- Water (1 cup): To mix and hydrate.

Instructions:

1. Mix the dandelion root and lemon juice in a cup of warm water.
2. Add honey and stir until dissolved.

- Drink slowly in the morning or before meals to support gallbladder health and detoxification.
- Freshly prepare each time, as it's best consumed right after mixing.

Rejuvelac for Digestive Wellness

Rejuvelac is a fermented drink made from sprouted grains, typically wheat, rye, or barley. It's rich in probiotics, which support gut health and can help heal leaky gut by promoting the growth of beneficial bacteria. The fermentation process produces lactic acid, enzymes, and vitamins that aid in digestion and improve the overall health of the gut lining.

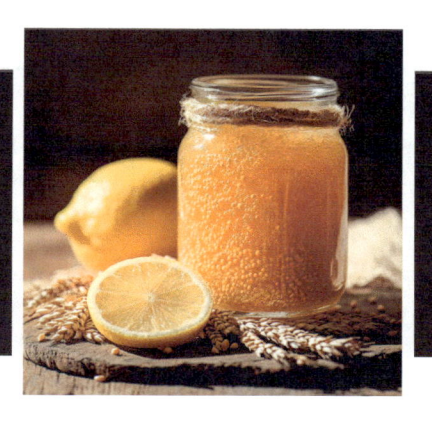

Ingredients:

- Sprouted Wheat, Rye, or Barley (1/2 cup): Acts as the base for fermentation, providing beneficial bacteria.
- Filtered Water (4 cups): Helps in fermenting the grains and infusing their nutrients.
- Optional: Lemon or Ginger (for flavor): Adds additional digestive support and a refreshing taste.

Instructions:

1. Rinse and soak the sprouted grains for 12-24 hours.
2. Place the grains in a large jar and cover with filtered water.
3. Cover the jar with a cloth and let it ferment at room temperature for 2-3 days.
4. Strain out the grains, and the liquid that remains is your Rejuvelac.

- Drink 1/4 to 1/2 cup of Rejuvelac daily to support gut health and promote healing of the intestinal lining.
- Store in the refrigerator for up to 1 week, and make fresh batches regularly.

Gut Health Morning Shots

This invigorating morning shot is designed to support gut health and kickstart digestion. With the powerful combination of ginger, lemon, and apple cider vinegar, this tonic helps to balance the gut, reduce bloating, and improve overall digestion.

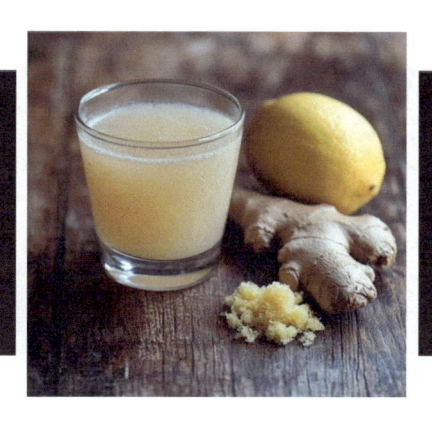

Ingredients:

- Ginger (1 teaspoon, grated): Known for its anti-inflammatory properties and ability to stimulate digestion.
- Lemon Juice (juice of 1 lemon): Boosts the immune system and supports liver detoxification.
- Apple Cider Vinegar (1 tablespoon): Supports gut health by promoting a healthy balance of stomach acids.
- Water (1/2 cup): Helps dilute and mix the ingredients.

Instructions:

1. Mix the ginger, lemon juice, and apple cider vinegar in a glass of water.
2. Stir well until fully combined.

- Drink this shot first thing in the morning to promote digestion and gut health.
- Freshly prepare each time, as it's best consumed right after mixing.

Herbal Acid Reflux Reliever

This soothing herbal tonic is designed to relieve the discomfort of acid reflux and support digestion. Crafted with ingredients known for their ability to balance stomach acidity and soothe the digestive tract, this remedy can help reduce symptoms like heartburn and indigestion.

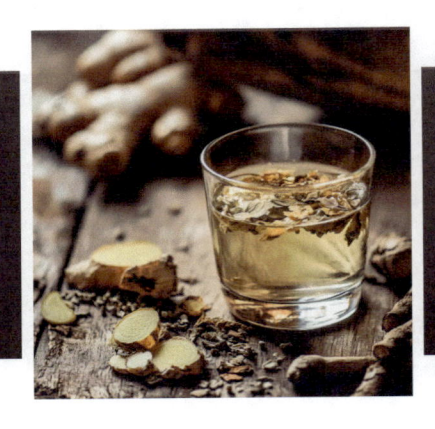

Ingredients:

- Slippery Elm (1 tablespoon): Known for its mucilage, which coats and soothes the digestive tract, reducing irritation caused by acid reflux.
- Marshmallow Root (1 tablespoon): Helps protect the mucous membranes of the stomach and esophagus, providing relief from acid reflux.
- Ginger (1 teaspoon, fresh or dried): Eases nausea and promotes healthy digestion, reducing the likelihood of acid buildup.
- Licorice Root (1 teaspoon): Helps to balance stomach acid levels and soothe inflammation in the esophagus.
- Water (1 cup): To mix and hydrate.

Instructions:

1. Mix all ingredients in a glass of warm water.
2. Stir well until everything is combined.

- Sip slowly before or after meals to promote digestion and reduce acid reflux.
- Freshly prepare each time, as it's best consumed right after mixing.

Ulcer & Gastritis Relief Tea

This soothing herbal tea blend is specially crafted to provide relief from conditions like gastritis, colitis, and ulcers. The combination of herbs helps to reduce inflammation, soothe the digestive tract, and promote healing for better digestive health.

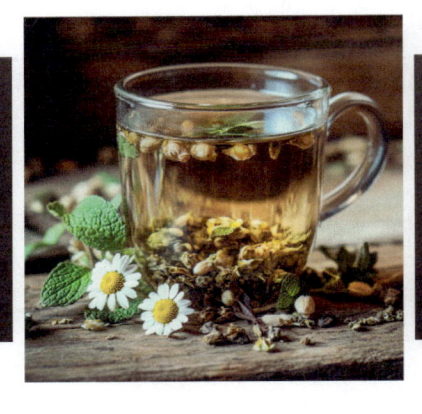

Ingredients:

- Chamomile (1 tablespoon): Known for its anti-inflammatory properties, chamomile helps calm the stomach and reduces irritation caused by gastritis and ulcers.
- Licorice Root (1 teaspoon): Helps protect and heal the stomach lining, reducing acid irritation and promoting digestion.
- Slippery Elm (1 tablespoon): Coats and soothes the mucous membranes of the digestive tract, offering relief from ulcers and gastritis.
- Marshmallow Root (1 tablespoon): Provides a protective coating to the stomach and intestines, reducing inflammation and promoting healing.
- Peppermint (1 teaspoon): Relieves gas, bloating, and discomfort, while soothing the digestive system.
- Water (1 cup): To mix and hydrate.

Instructions:

1. Mix all ingredients in a glass of warm water.
2. Stir well until everything is combined.

- Sip slowly before or after meals to soothe the digestive tract and alleviate symptoms of gastritis, colitis, and ulcers.
- Freshly prepare each time, as it's best consumed right after mixing.

Bowel Balance Elixir

This soothing elixir is crafted to help maintain healthy digestion and promote regular bowel movements. It combines natural ingredients that ease constipation, reduce bloating, and support overall digestive wellness.

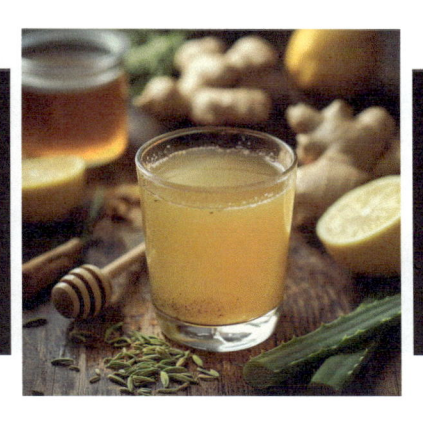

Ingredients:

- Aloe Vera Juice (2 tablespoons): Known for its soothing properties, aloe vera helps to calm the digestive tract and promotes regular bowel movements.
- Fennel Seeds (1 teaspoon): Fennel is widely used to reduce bloating and gas, aiding in digestion.
- Ginger (1 teaspoon, grated): Helps stimulate digestion and relieve discomfort from bloating and constipation.
- Lemon Juice (juice of 1 lemon): Aids digestion and detoxification, promoting a healthy bowel movement.
- Honey (1 teaspoon): Offers soothing properties and balances the flavors of the elixir.

Instructions:

1. Mix all ingredients in a glass of warm water.
2. Stir well until honey dissolves.

- Sip slowly in the morning or before meals to support healthy digestion and relieve constipation.
- Freshly prepare each time, as it's best consumed right after mixing.

Anti-Parasitic Black Walnut Drops

These Black Walnut drops are designed to help combat parasites and support a healthy digestive system. Known for their potent properties, black walnut hulls have been traditionally used to create an inhospitable environment for parasites while supporting intestinal health.

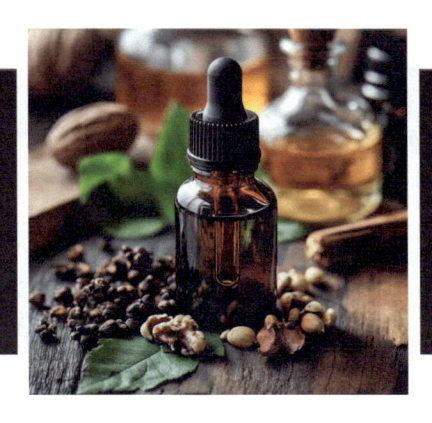

Ingredients:

- Black Walnut Hulls (1 tablespoon, powdered or finely chopped): Known for their anti-parasitic and astringent properties, helping eliminate parasites and cleanse the digestive system.
- Cloves (1 teaspoon, powdered): Contain eugenol, which is effective against parasites and helps maintain gut health.
- Filtered Water (1/2 cup): Used to dilute the extract.
- Apple Cider Vinegar (1/2 cup): Acts as a solvent to draw out the active compounds and enhance the digestive benefits.

Instructions:

1. Combine black walnut hulls and cloves in a clean jar.
2. Add apple cider vinegar and filtered water, ensuring the herbs are covered.
3. Seal and store in a cool, dark place for 2-3 weeks, shaking daily.
4. Strain and transfer the tincture to a dropper bottle.

- Take 10-15 drops daily for a limited period, ideally in the morning, to support digestive health.
- Store the tincture in a cool, dark place for up to 6 months.

Nature's Laxative Blend

This gentle, natural blend combines herbs known for their ability to support healthy digestion and relieve constipation without harsh side effects. A soothing and effective solution for promoting regularity.

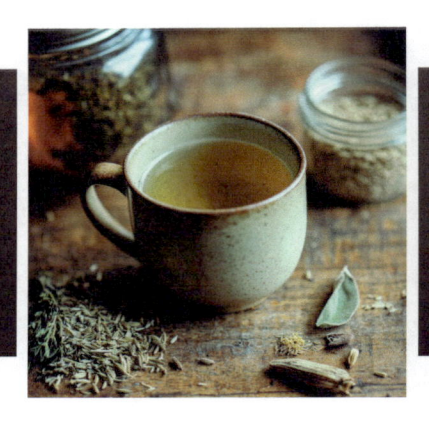

Ingredients:

- Senna Leaf (1 tablespoon, dried): A well-known natural laxative that promotes bowel movements by stimulating the muscles of the intestines.
- Cascara Sagrada (1 teaspoon, dried): Often used to stimulate bowel movements by promoting peristalsis and supporting overall colon health.
- Psyllium Husk (1 tablespoon): High in soluble fiber, it helps soften stool and promote healthy digestion.
- Fennel Seed (1 teaspoon, crushed): Known for its soothing properties, fennel aids digestion and can help relieve bloating and gas.
- Water (1 cup): To create an infusion and hydrate.

Instructions:

1. Mix the senna leaf, cascara sagrada, psyllium husk, and fennel seeds in a cup.
2. Pour 1 cup of hot water over the herbs and steep for 10-15 minutes.
3. Strain the herbs and drink the infusion warm.

- Sip slowly before bedtime to promote regularity and digestive comfort.
- Freshly prepare each time, as it's best consumed right after mixing.

Homemade Colon Detox Shot

This powerful detox shot combines ingredients that help cleanse the colon, promote healthy digestion, and eliminate waste, leaving your digestive system refreshed.

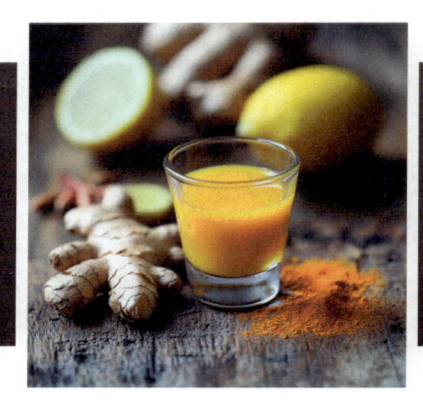

Ingredients:

- Lemon Juice (juice of 1 lemon): Rich in vitamin C, it stimulates bile production and promotes detoxification.
- Apple Cider Vinegar (1 tablespoon): Known for its ability to support digestion, balance pH, and stimulate detox processes.
- Ginger Root (1 teaspoon, grated): Soothes the digestive system, reduces inflammation, and promotes bowel movements.
- Turmeric (1/2 teaspoon): A powerful anti-inflammatory, it supports overall gut health and detoxifies the colon.
- Cayenne Pepper (a pinch): Boosts circulation and metabolism, helping to eliminate toxins and promote bowel regularity.
- Water (1/2 cup): To dilute and hydrate.

Instructions:

1. Mix all ingredients in a glass of warm water.
2. Stir well until everything is fully dissolved.

- Drink the shot in the morning on an empty stomach to jumpstart digestion and support colon detoxification.
- Freshly prepare each time, as it's best consumed right after mixing.

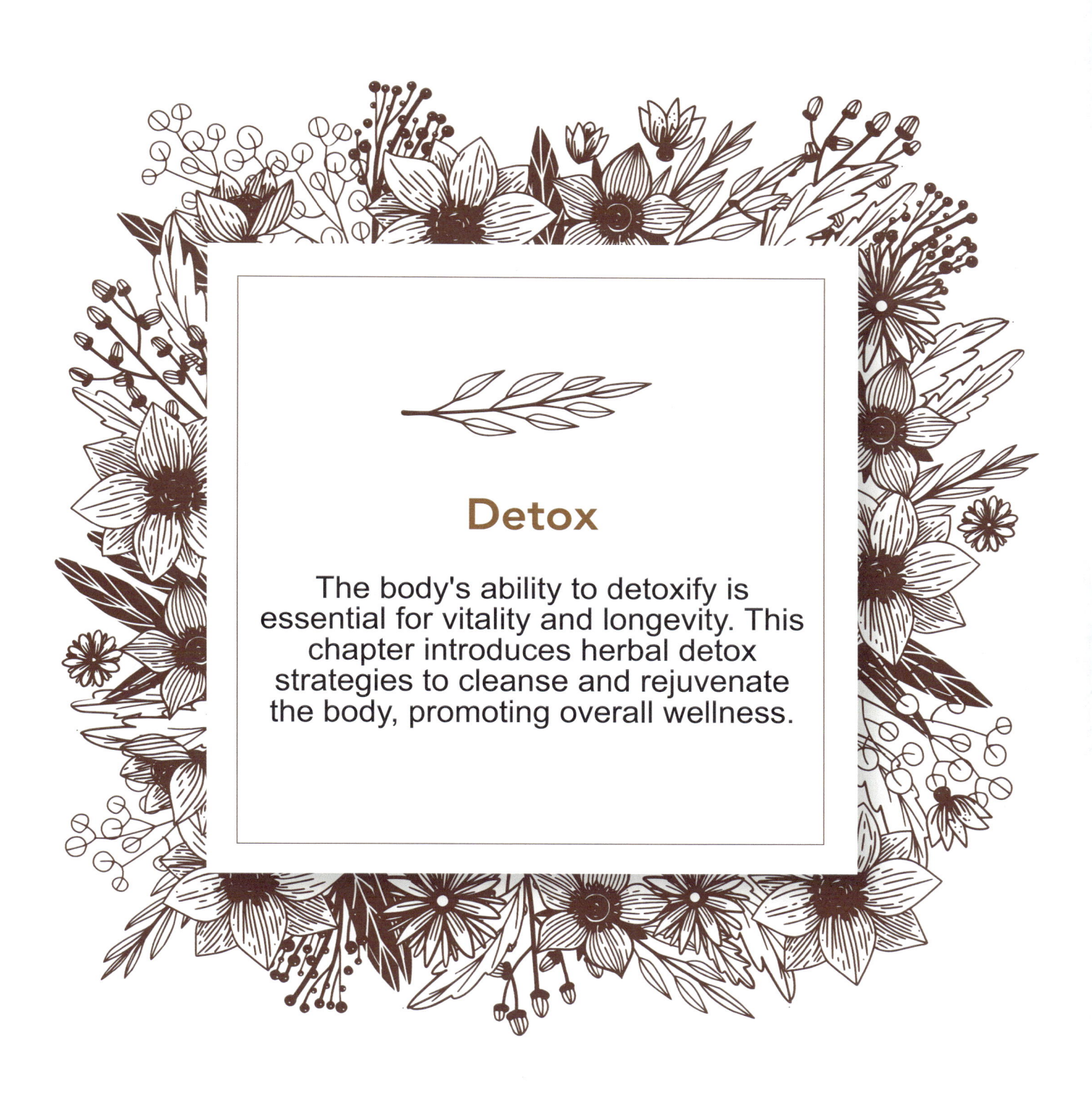

Detox

The body's ability to detoxify is essential for vitality and longevity. This chapter introduces herbal detox strategies to cleanse and rejuvenate the body, promoting overall wellness.

Bay Leaf Water

Bay leaf water is a simple herbal infusion known for its digestive benefits, anti-inflammatory properties, and potential to help regulate blood sugar levels. This gentle tea can be used as a daily wellness tonic.

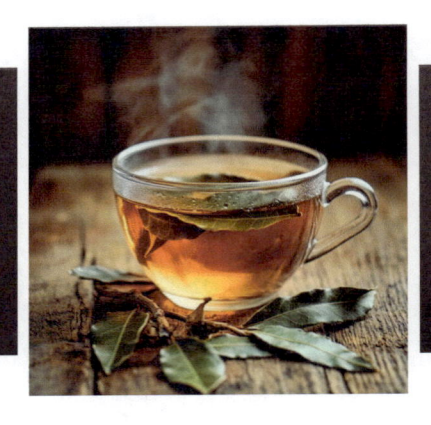

Ingredients:

- Bay Leaves (5-6 fresh or dried): Known for their antioxidants, aiding digestion, and reducing inflammation.
- Water (2 cups)

Instructions:

1. Bring water to a boil in a small pot.
2. Add bay leaves, reduce to a simmer, and let it steep for 5-10 minutes.
3. Strain the leaves and pour the infused water into a cup.

- Drink a cup on an empty stomach or after meals to support digestion. Enjoy up to two cups daily.
- Best enjoyed fresh, but can be stored in the fridge for up to a day.

Flat Tummy Capsules

These herbal capsules support digestion and may help reduce bloating. They incorporate natural herbs known for their soothing effects on the digestive system, making them ideal for supporting a flatter tummy and better digestive health.

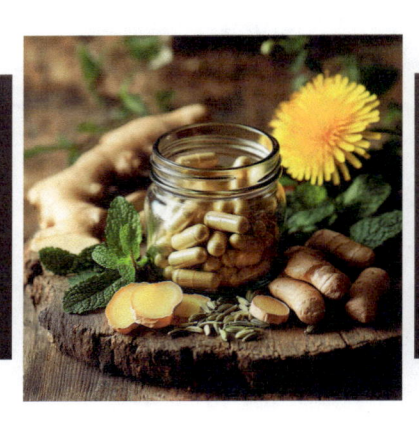

Ingredients:

- Dandelion Root Powder (1 teaspoon): Known for its gentle diuretic properties and ability to reduce water retention.
- Ginger Powder (1 teaspoon): Supports digestion and relieves bloating.
- Peppermint Leaf Powder (1 teaspoon): Soothes the stomach and helps ease gas.
- Fennel Seed Powder (1 teaspoon): Assists digestion and reduces bloating.
- Vegetable Capsules (Empty, approx. 30)

Instructions:

1. In a bowl, mix all the powders until well-blended.
2. Carefully fill each capsule with the powder mixture using a capsule filler or by hand.
3. Store the capsules in an airtight container.

- Take one capsule daily with a glass of water, preferably before a meal, to support digestion.
- Keep in a cool, dry place.

Craving Buster Brew

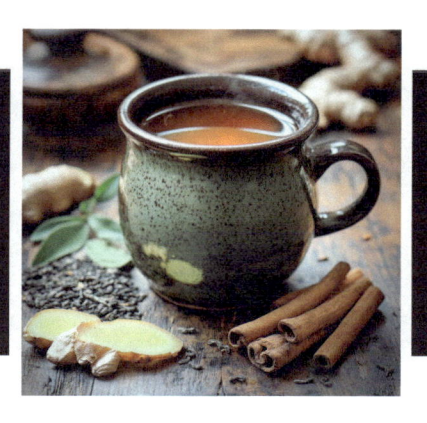

This herbal blend is designed to help curb cravings and promote balanced energy levels throughout the day. It combines herbs traditionally known for their appetite-suppressing properties and supportive effects on metabolism.

Ingredients:

- Green Tea (1 teaspoon): Provides gentle energy and helps reduce cravings by supporting metabolism.
- Fenugreek Seeds (1/2 teaspoon): Known to reduce appetite and support blood sugar balance.
- Cinnamon Powder (1/4 teaspoon): Helps stabilize blood sugar levels, reducing the likelihood of sudden cravings.
- Licorice Root (1/4 teaspoon): A naturally sweet herb that may help satisfy sugar cravings.
- Ginger Powder (1/4 teaspoon): Supports digestion and can help manage appetite.

Instructions:

1. Boil 2 cups of water in a saucepan.
2. Add all the herbs and let simmer on low for 10 minutes.
3. Strain and pour into a mug.

- Enjoy a cup mid-morning or in the afternoon to help manage cravings. Limit to 1-2 servings per day.
- Store unused dried ingredients in a cool, dry place.

Dandelion and Burdock Purge

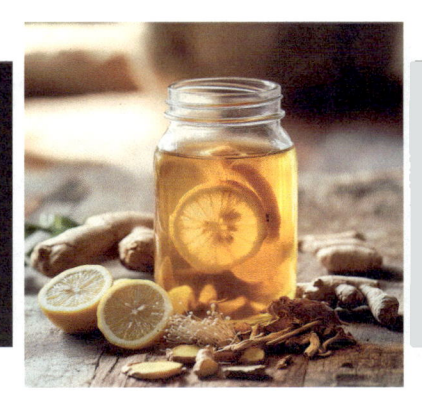

A natural herbal tonic made with dandelion and burdock, traditionally used to support liver health and assist in gentle detoxification.

Ingredients:

- Dandelion Root (1 tablespoon): Known for its cleansing properties, supports liver function and digestion.
- Burdock Root (1 tablespoon): Purifies the blood and aids in toxin removal.
- Ginger Root (1/2 teaspoon): Adds warmth, supports digestion, and may reduce nausea during detox.
- Fresh Lemon Juice (1 tablespoon): Rich in antioxidants, it aids in flushing out toxins.
- Honey (optional, 1 teaspoon): To sweeten the tonic naturally.

Instructions:

1. Add dandelion, burdock, and ginger roots to 3 cups of boiling water.
2. Simmer on low for 15 minutes, then strain.
3. Add lemon juice and honey if desired.

- Drink 1 cup, up to 3 times daily for a week to support detox. Adjust serving frequency based on personal tolerance.
- Keep any unused tonic refrigerated for up to 2 days.

Metabolic Herbal Coffee

A warming herbal blend designed to support metabolism and provide natural energy without the jitters of traditional coffee.

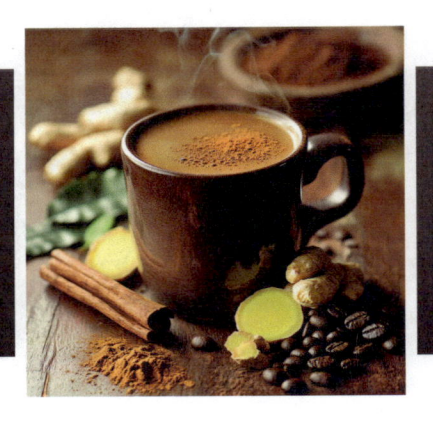

Ingredients:

- Green Coffee Bean Powder (1 tablespoon): Contains chlorogenic acids that may aid in weight loss and boost metabolism.
- Cinnamon (1/2 teaspoon): Known for regulating blood sugar levels and boosting metabolism.
- Ginger (1/2 teaspoon): Stimulates digestion and helps with fat metabolism.
- Turmeric (1/4 teaspoon): Supports inflammation reduction and digestion.
- Cocoa Powder (1 tablespoon): Adds a rich, chocolatey flavor while supporting heart health.
- Honey or Stevia (optional): For natural sweetness, if desired.

Instructions:

1. In a small pot, bring 1 cup of water to a boil.
2. Add all herbs and powders, stirring to combine.
3. Reduce heat and simmer for 5–10 minutes, allowing the herbs to infuse.
4. Strain into a mug and add honey or stevia if desired.
- Drink 1–2 cups per day, preferably in the morning, to support metabolic function and provide energy.
- Keep the herbal blend in an airtight container for up to 2 weeks.

Green Burn Smoothie

This nutrient-packed green smoothie is designed to support metabolism, detoxify the body, and help with weight management. The ingredients are carefully chosen for their ability to boost energy, curb cravings, and aid digestion.

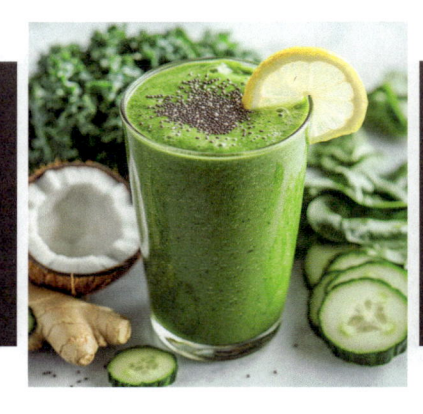

Ingredients:

- Spinach (1 cup): Rich in vitamins, minerals, and fiber, supporting digestion and metabolism.
- Kale (1/2 cup): High in antioxidants and supports detoxification.
- Green Apple (1): Adds natural sweetness and fiber, helping with digestion and cravings.
- Ginger (1 teaspoon): Aids digestion.
- Cucumber (1/2): Supports detoxification.
- Lemon Juice (1 tablespoon): Promotes digestion and helps alkalize the body.
- Chia Seeds (1 tablespoon): Packed with fiber and omega-3 fatty acids, supporting digestion.
- Coconut Water (1 cup): Provides hydration and electrolytes.
- Stevia or Honey (optional): For sweetness, if desired.

Instructions:

1. Combine all ingredients in a blender.
2. Blend until smooth, adding coconut water to adjust the consistency as needed.
3. Serve immediately and enjoy.

- Drink 1-2 times a day to boost metabolism, support digestion, and assist with weight management.
- Best consumed fresh but can be stored in the fridge for up to 24 hours.

Forskolin Capsules to Boost Metabolism

Forskolin, derived from the root of the Coleus forskohlii plant, has been traditionally used in Ayurvedic medicine. It is believed to help in boosting metabolism by increasing levels of cyclic AMP (cAMP) in the body, which can stimulate fat-burning and support weight management.

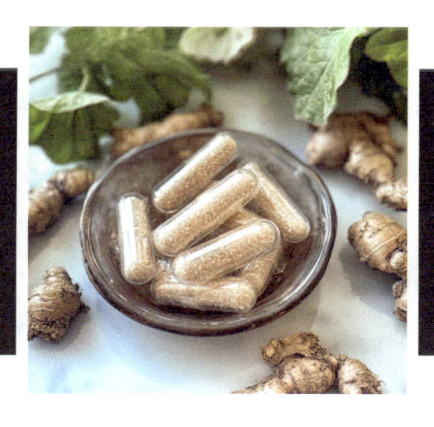

Ingredients:

- Forskolin Root Powder (500 mg): The main ingredient that is believed to enhance fat loss by activating enzymes that break down stored fat.
- Gelatin Capsules: To encapsulate the forskolin powder for easy ingestion.

Instructions:

1. Measure 500 mg of forskolin root powder.
2. Fill the gelatin capsules with the powder using a capsule filling machine or by hand.
3. Seal the capsules and store them in a dark, cool place.
- Take 1-2 capsules daily, preferably before meals. Monitor your body's response and adjust the dosage if necessary.
- Store in a dry, cool place, away from direct sunlight.
- Note: While forskolin may support fat loss, it's important to combine it with a healthy diet and exercise for optimal results. Always consult with a healthcare provider before starting any supplement regimen, especially if you have existing health conditions.

Cleansing Stinging Nettle Soup

To simplify the Cleansing Stinging Nettle Soup, you can remove or substitute certain ingredients. Here's a modified version with fewer ingredients while still keeping it effective:

Ingredients:

- Olive Oil (2 tbsp): Retain for healthy fats and flavor.
- Onion (1, chopped): Keep for flavor and digestive support.
- Vegetable Broth (4 cups): Essential for hydration and as the soup's base.
- Fresh Stinging Nettle Leaves (2–3 cups): The main detoxifying ingredient.
- Potato (1, peeled and diced): Optional, but adds texture. You can also skip it if you want a lighter version.
- Salt & Pepper: For basic seasoning.

Instructions:

1. Rinse the nettles and set aside.
2. Heat olive oil in a pot, sauté the onion until softened.
3. Add vegetable broth and diced potato (if using) and simmer for 15-20 minutes.
4. Stir in nettles and let cook for 5-10 minutes.
5. Blend the soup to a smooth texture and season with salt and pepper.

- Enjoy 1–2 servings per week for detox support.
- Refrigerate for 3 days or freeze for longer storage.

Metabolic Superfood Bars

These simple yet effective bars are designed to support metabolism and energy levels. With just a few wholesome ingredients, they provide a convenient and delicious way to stay nourished while aiding digestion and promoting a healthy metabolism.

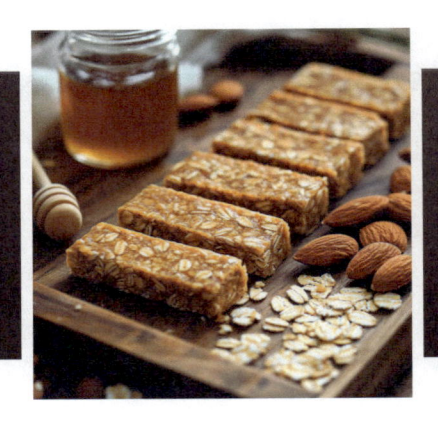

Ingredients:

- Almonds (1/2 cup): Rich in healthy fats and protein, almonds help stabilize blood sugar and boost metabolism.
- Oats (1/2 cup): Full of fiber, oats promote digestion and provide steady energy throughout the day.
- Coconut Oil (2 tbsp): Contains healthy fats that support fat metabolism and energy.
- Honey or Maple Syrup (2 tbsp): Natural sweeteners that provide a quick energy source and help bind the ingredients together.
- Cinnamon (1/2 tsp): Known to regulate blood sugar and support metabolism.

Instructions:

1. Preheat the oven to 350°F (175°C).
2. Mix all dry ingredients (almonds, oats, cinnamon) in a bowl.
3. Stir in the wet ingredients (coconut oil and honey/maple syrup) and combine thoroughly.
4. Press the mixture into a lined baking dish and bake for 15–20 minutes until firm and golden.
5. Allow to cool before cutting into bars.
- Enjoy a bar as a snack or part of your breakfast to support your metabolism.
- These bars offer an easy way to boost your metabolism with minimal ingredients and maximum health benefits.

All-Day Slimming Tea

A gentle blend of herbs known for aiding digestion, boosting metabolism, and supporting detox, this tea can be enjoyed throughout the day to help with slimming goals in a natural way.

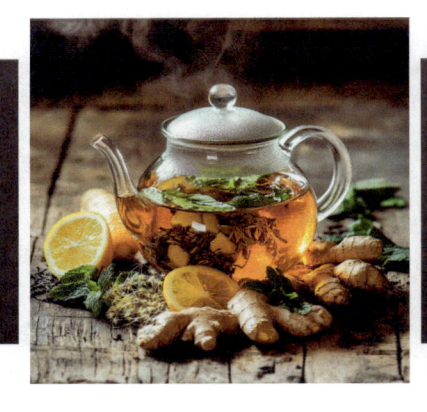

Ingredients:

- Green Tea (1 teaspoon): Boosts metabolism and provides antioxidants.
- Ginger Root (1-inch piece, sliced): Helps with digestion and adds a warm flavor.
- Dandelion Root (1 teaspoon, dried): Supports liver health and natural detoxification.
- Peppermint (1 teaspoon, dried): Soothes digestion and provides a refreshing flavor.
- Lemon Peel (1 teaspoon, dried): Adds vitamin C and supports metabolism.
-

Instructions:

1. Combine all ingredients in a teapot or infuser.
2. Pour 2 cups of hot water over the herbs and let steep for 5-7 minutes.
3. Strain and enjoy hot or cold, sipping throughout the day.

- Drink 2-3 cups daily, spaced out during the day, for a gentle slimming effect.
- Store dried herbs in a cool, dry place and prepare fresh each day for best results.

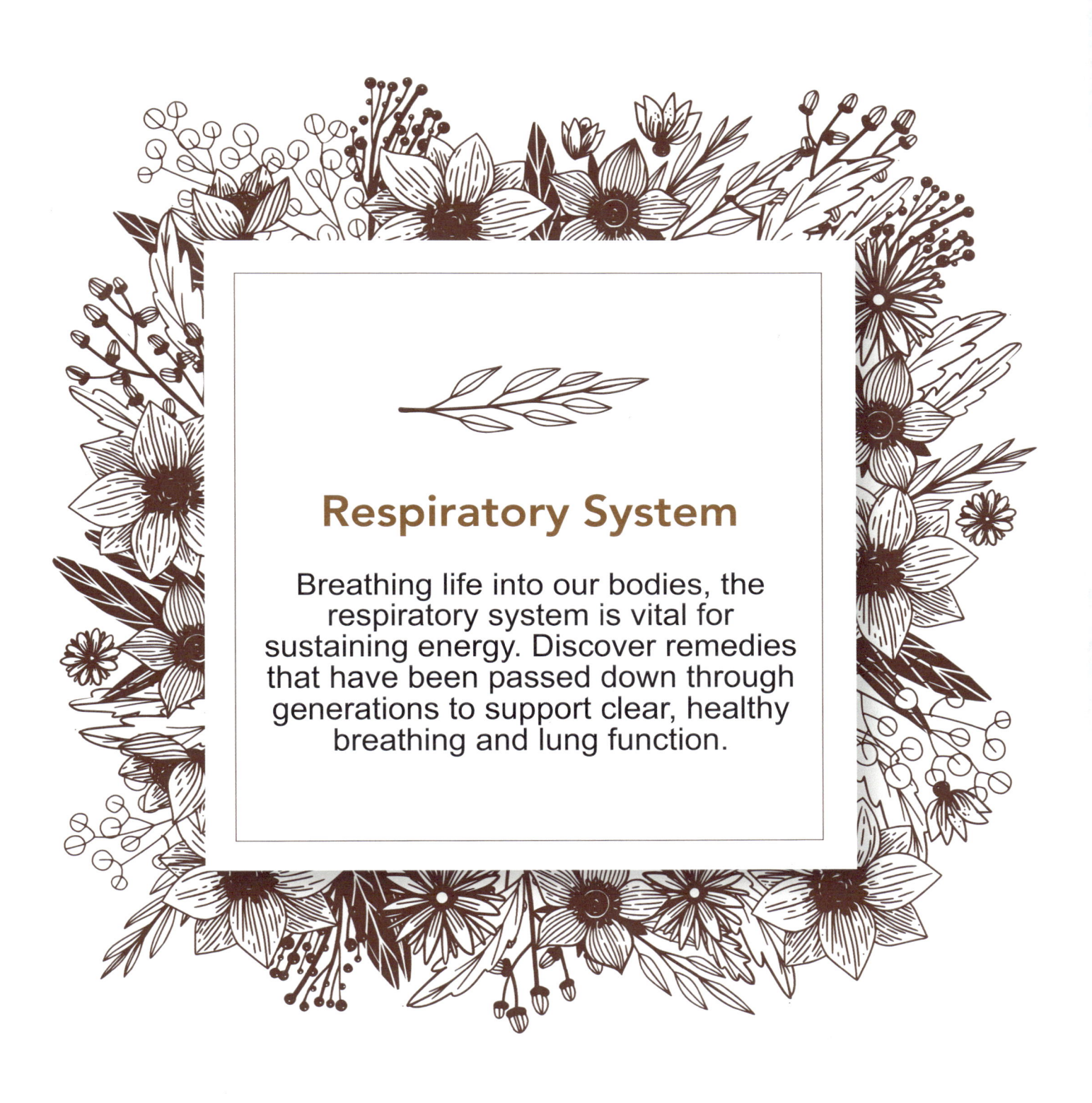

Respiratory System

Breathing life into our bodies, the respiratory system is vital for sustaining energy. Discover remedies that have been passed down through generations to support clear, healthy breathing and lung function.

Mullein and Marshmallow Cough Syrup

This natural cough syrup combines the soothing and anti-inflammatory properties of mullein and marshmallow root, two herbs traditionally used to ease coughing, sore throat, and respiratory discomfort. It's a gentle and effective way to support throat and lung health.

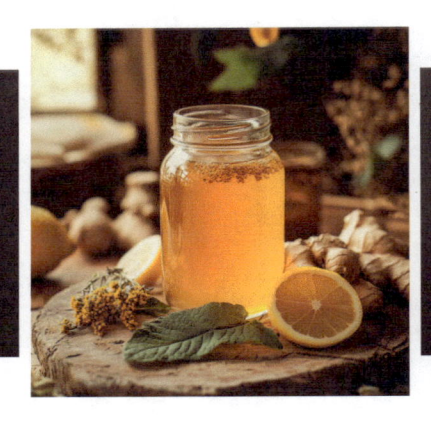

Ingredients:

- Mullein (1 tablespoon, dried): Known for its soothing properties on the respiratory tract, helping to reduce irritation and inflammation.
- Marshmallow Root (1 tablespoon, dried): A mucilaginous herb that coats the throat, providing relief from irritation and helping to ease coughing.
- Honey (1/2 cup): Offers natural antibacterial properties and soothes the throat.
- Apple Cider Vinegar (2 tablespoons): Helps to thin mucus and clear congestion.
- Lemon Juice (2 tablespoons): Provides vitamin C and helps to cut through mucus.
- Ginger (1 teaspoon, grated): Adds a warming effect and helps soothe irritation in the throat.

Instructions:

1. Combine the mullein and marshmallow root with 2 cups of water in a saucepan.
2. Bring to a simmer, and let it steep for 15-20 minutes.
3. Strain the herbs out, and return the liquid to the saucepan.
4. Stir in honey, apple cider vinegar, lemon juice, and ginger. Heat gently until everything is combined.
5. Pour the syrup into a clean jar or bottle and let it cool.
- Take 1 tablespoon every 2-3 hours as needed for relief from coughing and throat irritation.

Rosemary and Sage Sore Throat Spray

This soothing herbal spray combines the antibacterial and anti-inflammatory properties of rosemary and sage to help relieve the discomfort of a sore throat. Both herbs have been traditionally used to combat throat infections and ease irritation, while providing natural relief without harsh chemicals.

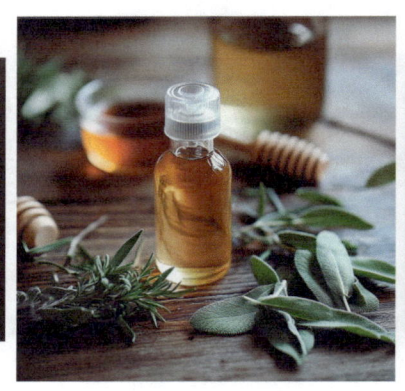

Ingredients:

- Rosemary (1 tablespoon): Known for its antimicrobial properties, rosemary helps to reduce throat inflammation and infection.
- Sage (1 tablespoon): Traditionally used to treat sore throats, sage has antiseptic qualities and can help relieve pain and irritation.
- Apple Cider Vinegar (1/4 cup): Helps balance pH and provides additional antimicrobial benefits.
- Filtered Water (1/2 cup): Acts as the base for the spray.
- Honey (1 tablespoon): Adds a soothing effect and natural sweetness, helping to coat the throat and reduce irritation.

Instructions:

1. Boil the water and steep rosemary and sage leaves in it for 10 minutes to make an herbal infusion.
2. Strain the herbs out of the liquid and let the infusion cool to room temperature.
3. Add apple cider vinegar and honey to the cooled infusion.
4. Pour the mixture into a small spray bottle and shake well before each use.
- Spray the solution into your throat as needed for relief, especially before meals or before bed. You can use it several times a day.
- Store the spray in the refrigerator for up to 1 week. Make sure to shake before each use.

Honey Lemon Ginger Cough Drops

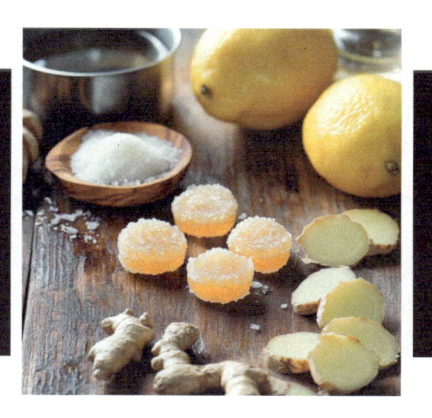

These homemade cough drops are a natural remedy to soothe a sore throat and alleviate coughing. Honey coats the throat, lemon provides vitamin C, and ginger helps with inflammation, making this an easy and effective solution.

Ingredients:

- Honey (1/4 cup): Soothes and coats the throat, has antibacterial properties.
- Lemon Juice (2 tablespoons): Packed with vitamin C to boost immunity and help clear mucus.
- Ginger Root (1 teaspoon, grated): Helps reduce inflammation and throat irritation.
- Coconut Oil (1 tablespoon): Binds the ingredients together for a smooth texture.
- Filtered Water (1/4 cup): Thin the mixture.
- Optional: Cornstarch (1/2 tablespoon): Helps create a firmer texture for the drops.

Instructions:

1. Combine honey, lemon juice, and grated ginger in a saucepan.
2. Add water and heat on low for 5-10 minutes, stirring regularly.
3. Once it thickens, remove from heat and stir in coconut oil and cornstarch (if using).
4. Pour into molds or spread on a baking sheet and let cool for 30 minutes.
5. Break into individual drops once firm.
- Suck on one drop as needed for relief from coughing or a sore throat.
- Keep in an airtight container at room temperature for up to 2 weeks.

Mustard Plaster

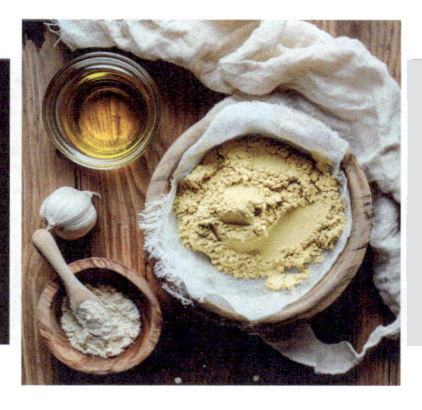

Mustard plaster is a traditional remedy used to relieve chest congestion, muscle pain, and inflammation. The heat from the mustard seeds can stimulate circulation and help loosen mucus, while their natural properties support respiratory health.

Ingredients:

- Mustard Powder (1/4 cup): Stimulates circulation and can help break down congestion in the chest.
- Flour (1/4 cup): Helps form the paste and reduces the intensity of the mustard's heat.
- Water (1-2 tablespoons): To form a paste with the mustard powder.
- Olive Oil or Coconut Oil (1 tablespoon): Adds moisture and helps protect the skin from irritation.
- Cheesecloth or Cloth (for wrapping the plaster)

Instructions:

1. In a bowl, mix mustard powder and flour.
2. Slowly add water, stirring until a thick paste forms.
3. Add oil to the paste and mix well.
4. Spread the mixture onto a piece of cheesecloth or a clean cloth.
5. Apply the plaster to the chest or the affected area. Ensure the mustard is not too hot to avoid burns.
6. Leave it on for 10-15 minutes, then remove and wash the area with warm water.
- Use once or twice a day as needed for congestion or muscle pain. Always check the skin for irritation after removal.
- Mustard paste is best used fresh but can be stored in a sealed container for up to a week.

Heating Potato Pad

A heating potato pad is a simple, natural way to soothe sore muscles, cramps, and inflammation. Potatoes retain heat well, making them an excellent choice for creating a homemade compress that can provide comfort and pain relief.

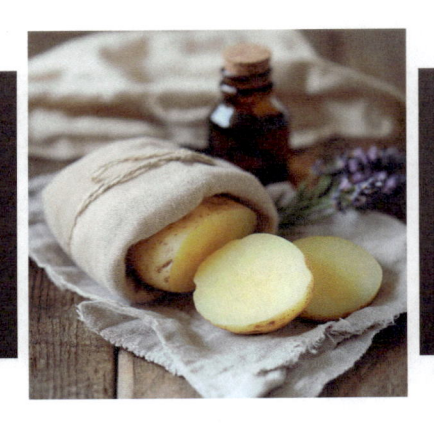

Ingredients:

- 1 large potato: Known for its heat-retaining properties.
- Clean cloth or cotton sock: To wrap the potato and hold the heat in.
- Optional: Essential oils (lavender, peppermint): For added soothing benefits.

Instructions:

1. Wash and peel the potato, then cut it into thin slices or mash it slightly (depending on your preference).
2. Wrap the potato slices or mashed potato in a clean cloth or a cotton sock.
3. Microwave the wrapped potato for 1-2 minutes, or heat it on a stovetop for a few minutes until warm (not too hot to avoid burns).
- Apply the heated potato pad to sore muscles, cramps, or inflamed areas. Use for 10-15 minutes, making sure the heat remains tolerable.
- Discard after each use. You can make a fresh one as needed.

Amish Cough Syrup

This traditional Amish cough syrup is made from simple, natural ingredients known for their soothing and healing properties. It is a natural remedy to help alleviate coughing, sore throat, and congestion.

Ingredients:

- Raw Honey (1 cup): Known for its antimicrobial properties and soothing effect on the throat.
- Apple Cider Vinegar (1/4 cup): Helps thin mucus and promotes respiratory health.
- Lemon Juice (2 tablespoons): Rich in vitamin C and helps to clear out mucus.
- Ginger (1 tablespoon, freshly grated): Acts as a natural anti-inflammatory and helps soothe the throat.
- Garlic (1-2 cloves, minced): Known for its natural antibiotic and immune-boosting properties.
- Cayenne Pepper (1/4 teaspoon, optional): Adds warmth and may help clear congestion.

Instructions:

1. In a saucepan, combine the honey, apple cider vinegar, and lemon juice. Gently heat over low heat until warm.
2. Add the grated ginger, garlic, and cayenne pepper if using. Stir to combine.
3. Let the mixture steep for 10-15 minutes.
4. Strain the syrup if desired, then store it in a glass jar or bottle.
- Take 1 tablespoon of the syrup every few hours as needed to soothe coughing and support throat health.

Sinus Relief Eucalyptus Steam

This eucalyptus steam remedy provides a natural way to clear sinuses, relieve congestion, and promote easier breathing. The steam opens up nasal passages, while the eucalyptus oil offers anti-inflammatory and antimicrobial properties.

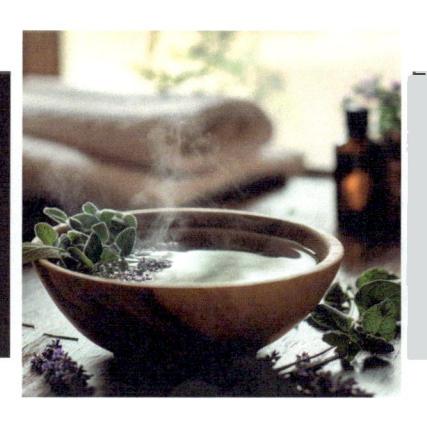

Ingredients:

- Eucalyptus Essential Oil (5-10 drops): Known for its ability to clear nasal congestion and its soothing, antimicrobial properties.
- Hot Water (1 bowl or pot): Used to generate the steam.
- Peppermint Essential Oil (optional, 3-5 drops): Adds a cooling effect and supports deeper breathing.
- Lavender Essential Oil (optional, 3-5 drops): Provides calming and anti-inflammatory properties to soothe irritation in the sinuses.

Instructions:

1. Boil water and pour it into a heatproof bowl or basin.
2. Add eucalyptus essential oil to the hot water.
3. (Optional) Add peppermint and lavender oils to enhance the experience.
4. Place a towel over your head and the bowl to trap the steam, and lean over the bowl, breathing deeply through your nose.
5. Steam for 5-10 minutes, making sure to take breaks if needed.
- Perform this steam inhalation 1-2 times a day when feeling congested or needing sinus relief.
- Use fresh each time; do not store the steam solution.

Hot Herbal Compress for Sinus Infection Relief

This hot herbal compress is designed to soothe sinus pressure, alleviate discomfort, and promote drainage. Warmth from the compress helps increase circulation, while the herbs provide natural decongestant and antimicrobial benefits.

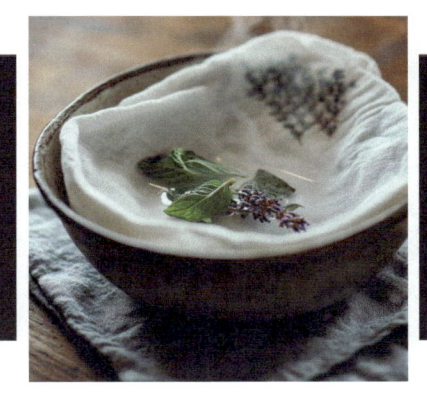

Ingredients:

- Dried Eucalyptus (1 tablespoon): Helps relieve sinus congestion and has antimicrobial properties.
- Dried Peppermint (1 tablespoon): Provides a cooling sensation, aids in relieving sinus pressure, and clears nasal passages.
- Dried Lavender (optional, 1 tablespoon): Soothes inflammation and provides a calming effect.
- Clean Cotton Cloth or Muslin Bag

Instructions:

1. Boil a small pot of water and remove it from heat.
2. Place the dried herbs in a muslin bag or tie them in a clean cotton cloth.
3. Dip the herb-filled cloth in the hot water, letting it steep and absorb the warmth.
4. Allow the compress to cool to a comfortable temperature.
5. Place the warm compress over your sinus area (forehead, cheeks, or nose) for 10-15 minutes, breathing deeply.

- Repeat 1-2 times a day as needed for sinus relief.
- Prepare fresh each time for maximum effectiveness.

Herbal Gargle for Throat Infection Relief

This herbal gargle helps soothe sore throats and ease inflammation. Using natural antimicrobial and anti-inflammatory herbs, it provides relief and promotes healing for throat infections.

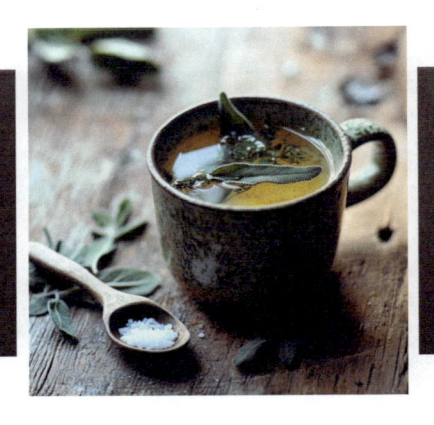

Ingredients:

- Salt (1/2 teaspoon): Helps reduce swelling and kill bacteria.
- Sage (1 teaspoon, dried or fresh): Antimicrobial and soothing for throat discomfort.
- Thyme (1/2 teaspoon): Has antibacterial and antifungal properties, aiding in infection relief.
- Honey (optional, 1/2 teaspoon): Provides soothing effects and natural sweetness.
- Warm Water (1 cup)

Instructions:

1. Boil water and pour it over the sage and thyme in a mug. Steep for 10 minutes, then strain.
2. Stir in the salt and honey (if using) until dissolved.
3. Gargle with the mixture for 30 seconds, then spit it out. Repeat until the cup is finished.

- Use 2–3 times a day for relief until symptoms subside.
- Prepare fresh for each use to retain potency.

Soothing Elixir for Cold and Flu Relief

This comforting elixir combines herbal ingredients known for their ability to ease cold and flu symptoms. It soothes sore throats, eases congestion, and provides a gentle energy boost to aid in recovery.

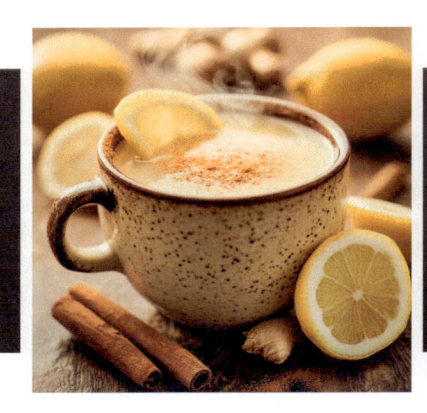

Ingredients:

- Honey (1 tablespoon): Soothes sore throats and provides antibacterial properties.
- Lemon Juice (1 tablespoon): High in vitamin C, it boosts immunity and supports hydration.
- Ginger (1 teaspoon, grated): Reduces inflammation, helps clear congestion, and warms the body.
- Cinnamon (1/4 teaspoon): Known for its warming effects and ability to reduce mucus.
- Warm Water (1 cup)

Instructions:

1. In a cup, combine honey, lemon juice, grated ginger, and cinnamon.
2. Pour warm water over the mixture, stirring until everything is well combined.
3. Let it sit for a minute, allowing the flavors to meld.

- Sip slowly throughout the day, especially during the morning and evening, for relief from cold and flu symptoms.
- Best made fresh before each use. If needed, refrigerate for up to 24 hours and reheat gently.

Grandma's Herbal Antibiotic

A natural, homemade remedy inspired by traditional herbal practices, this blend is meant to help support the body's natural defenses during mild infections. Ingredients are selected for their reputed antibacterial, antiviral, and immune-boosting properties.

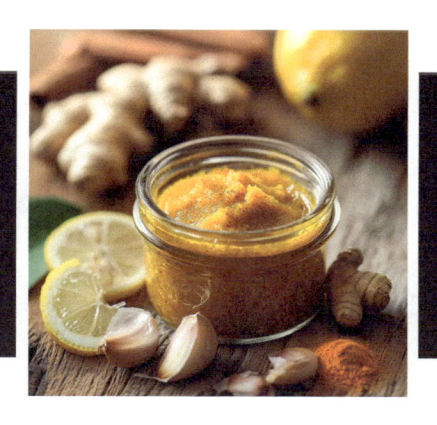

Ingredients:

- Garlic (1 clove, minced): Known for its powerful antibacterial and antiviral qualities.
- Raw Honey (1 tablespoon): Soothes and coats the throat while providing mild antibacterial support.
- Ginger (1/2 teaspoon, grated): Reduces inflammation and promotes immune function.
- Apple Cider Vinegar (1 tablespoon): Contains acetic acid, which may help fight bacteria and balance pH.
- Turmeric Powder (1/4 teaspoon): Offers anti-inflammatory and antimicrobial benefits.
- Lemon Juice (1 tablespoon): Provides vitamin C to support immunity.

Instructions:

1. In a small bowl, combine the minced garlic, honey, grated ginger, apple cider vinegar, turmeric, and lemon juice.
2. Stir until well-mixed and let sit for 5–10 minutes to allow flavors to meld.
3. Strain if desired, or consume as is for a stronger effect.

- Take 1–2 teaspoons daily when you feel early signs of a mild infection. Swallow slowly to coat the throat.
- Store in a glass jar in the refrigerator for up to 3 days. Shake before each use.

Homemade Rub for Easy Breathing

This soothing chest rub combines respiratory-supportive herbs and essential oils to help open nasal passages, ease congestion, and promote clear breathing. It's a natural alternative to commercial vapor rubs, providing a gentle yet effective remedy for easier breathing during colds and congestion.

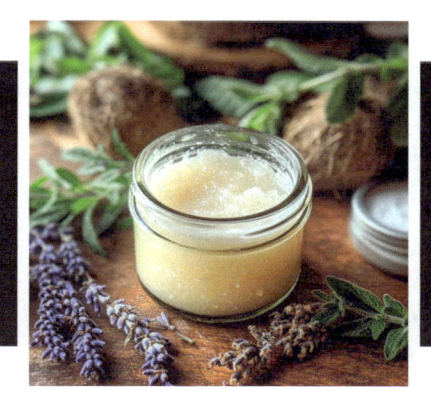

Ingredients:

- Coconut Oil (2 tablespoons): Acts as a moisturizing base for the rub.
- Beeswax (1 teaspoon): Helps thicken the rub to a balm consistency.
- Eucalyptus Essential Oil (5 drops): Known for its cooling, decongestant properties.
- Peppermint Essential Oil (5 drops): Opens up nasal passages and relieves stuffiness.
- Rosemary Essential Oil (3 drops): Provides a gentle warming effect and supports respiratory health.
- Lavender Essential Oil (3 drops): Soothes and calms, promoting relaxation.

Instructions:

1. In a double boiler, melt the coconut oil and beeswax until fully combined.
2. Remove from heat and let cool slightly before adding essential oils.
3. Stir well, then pour the mixture into a small container or jar and allow it to cool and solidify.

- Apply a small amount to the chest, neck, and back as needed. For best results, use before sleep or anytime you need breathing relief.
- Store in a cool, dry place for up to 6 months.

Breath-Ease Thyme Syrup

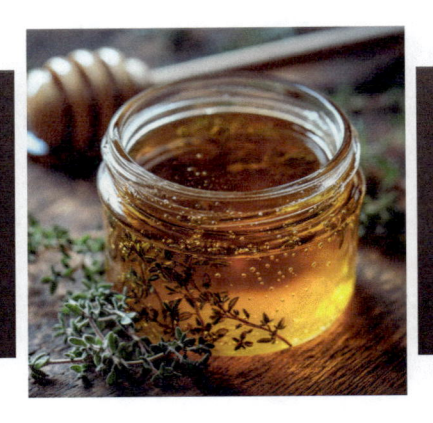

This herbal syrup combines thyme and honey to support respiratory health, soothe coughs, and ease congestion. Thyme has natural antimicrobial properties that can help alleviate respiratory discomfort, making it an ideal choice for colds, coughs, and other respiratory issues.

Ingredients:

- Fresh or Dried Thyme (1/2 cup): Known for its respiratory-supporting and antimicrobial properties.
- Water (1 cup): To extract the beneficial compounds from thyme.
- Honey (1/2 cup): Soothes the throat and acts as a natural preservative for the syrup.

Instructions:

1. In a saucepan, bring water to a gentle simmer, then add thyme.
2. Let simmer for about 15-20 minutes, then remove from heat and strain.
3. Once the liquid cools slightly, add honey and stir well.
4. Pour into a glass jar and refrigerate.

- Take 1-2 teaspoons as needed for cough relief or respiratory support.
- Store in the refrigerator for up to two weeks.

Lung Strength Drops

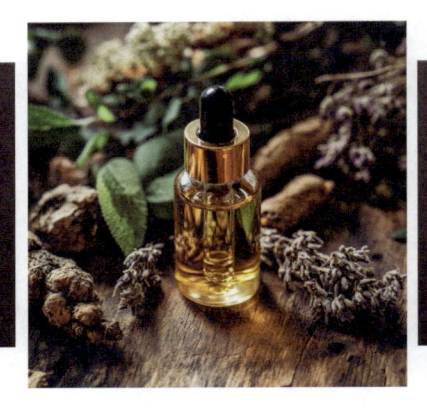

These herbal drops are crafted to support lung function and respiratory health. The selected ingredients work to soothe, clear, and strengthen the lungs, especially beneficial during seasonal changes or for general respiratory support.

Ingredients:

- Mullein Leaf (1 tablespoon, dried): Traditionally used to help soothe respiratory irritation and reduce mucus buildup.
- Elecampane Root (1 teaspoon, dried): Known for its lung-supporting properties, elecampane aids in clearing mucus and promoting healthy airflow.
- Thyme (1 teaspoon, dried): An herb with antimicrobial qualities that supports clear breathing and respiratory wellness.
- Filtered Water (1/2 cup): For infusion purposes.
- Apple Cider Vinegar (1/2 cup): Extracts active compounds from the herbs and enhances their respiratory benefits.

Instructions:

1. Combine mullein leaf, elecampane root, and thyme in a clean glass jar.
2. Add the apple cider vinegar and filtered water, making sure the herbs are fully submerged.
3. Seal and store in a cool, dark place for 2-3 weeks, shaking daily.
4. Strain the mixture and transfer it to a dropper bottle.

- Take 10-15 drops once or twice daily to support lung health, especially during times when respiratory support is needed.

Frontier Cough Soother

This natural remedy combines soothing herbs that are known for their ability to calm coughs, ease irritation, and support overall respiratory health. Ideal for those looking for a gentle yet effective solution to alleviate throat discomfort.

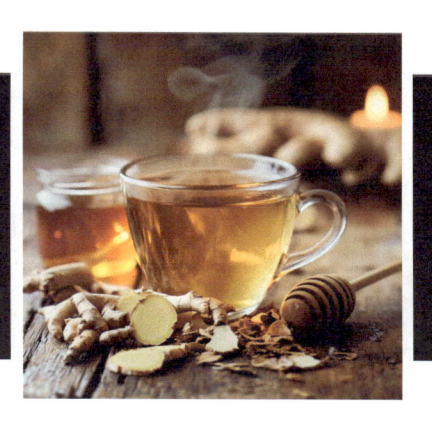

Ingredients:

- Marshmallow Root (1 tablespoon): Known for its mucilage content, it helps coat and soothe irritated tissues in the throat.
- Slippery Elm (1 tablespoon): Works similarly to marshmallow root, providing a protective layer for the throat and reducing irritation.
- Ginger (1 teaspoon): Adds warmth and promotes circulation, helping to relieve congestion and soothe coughs.
- Licorice Root (1/2 tablespoon): Supports the respiratory system and works as a mild expectorant.
- Honey (2 teaspoons): Naturally soothing and antimicrobial, honey helps coat the throat and reduce coughing.

Instructions:

1. Boil 2 cups of water and add the herbs.
2. Let simmer for 10-15 minutes, stirring occasionally.
3. Strain and pour the tea into a cup, adding honey to taste.

- Drink 1-2 cups per day when experiencing throat discomfort or coughing.
- Best consumed fresh. Store any leftover tea in the fridge for up to 24 hours.

Warm Comfort Brew

This cozy, soothing drink is perfect for calming your senses and warming you up on chilly days. Combining herbs known for their relaxing and anti-inflammatory properties, this brew helps to ease tension and promote comfort.

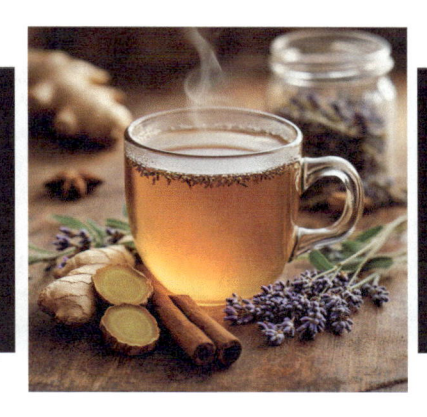

Ingredients:

- Chamomile (1 tablespoon): A calming herb that helps relax the body and mind, promoting a restful feeling.
- Lavender (1 teaspoon): Known for its calming and anti-inflammatory effects, it soothes tension and supports relaxation.
- Ginger (1 teaspoon): Adds warmth and helps improve circulation, soothing digestive discomforts.
- Cinnamon Stick (1): Adds a comforting spice that supports digestion and warms the body.
- Honey (1 tablespoon): Naturally soothing for the throat, honey adds sweetness and has mild antibacterial properties.

Instructions:

1. Boil 2 cups of water and add the chamomile, lavender, ginger, and cinnamon stick.
2. Let the mixture simmer for 10 minutes, allowing the flavors to meld together.
3. Strain into a mug and stir in honey to taste.

- Enjoy a warm cup in the evening or whenever you're in need of comfort and relaxation.
- Best consumed fresh, but can be stored in the fridge for up to 24 hours.

Jello Flu Shots

These homemade gel shots combine ingredients known for their immune-boosting and symptom-relieving properties. Perfect for those who struggle with taking pills or traditional liquid remedies, these shots provide a comforting, gelatinous form of relief.

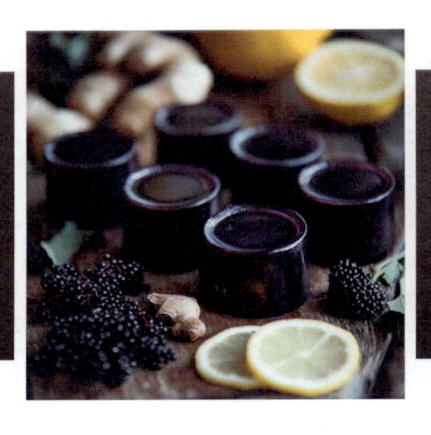

Ingredients:

- Elderberry Syrup (2 tbsp): Packed with antioxidants and immune-boosting compounds, elderberry can help reduce the severity and duration of flu symptoms.
- Honey (1 tbsp): Known for its soothing properties, honey helps calm a sore throat and has natural antibacterial benefits.
- Ginger (1 tbsp, grated): Offers anti-inflammatory effects and helps with nausea and digestive issues, often experienced during the flu.
- Gelatin (2 tbsp): The base for the "shots," providing a gel-like consistency for easy consumption.
- Lemon Juice (1 tbsp): High in vitamin C, lemon juice can support the immune system and help detoxify the body.

Instructions:

1. In a small saucepan, combine elderberry syrup, grated ginger, honey, and lemon juice. Warm gently over low heat, stirring frequently.
2. Once the ingredients are well combined, slowly stir in the gelatin until fully dissolved.
3. Pour the mixture into silicone molds or an ice cube tray for easy shot servings.
4. Allow the mixture to cool and set in the refrigerator for about 2 hours or until solid.
- Consume 1-2 "Jello Flu Shots" per day as needed to soothe flu symptoms.
- Keep the shots in an airtight container in the fridge for up to one week.

Clear Chest Basil Brew

This aromatic brew combines herbs known for their respiratory and anti-inflammatory properties. The basil and other soothing ingredients in this tea can help clear congestion and ease breathing difficulties, making it a comforting remedy for colds or chest discomfort.

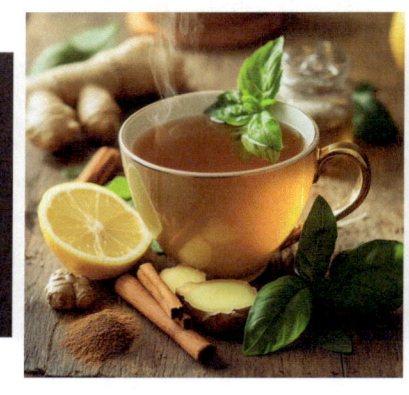

Ingredients:

- Basil Leaves (1/2 cup): Basil contains anti-inflammatory and antimicrobial properties that help clear the airways and reduce chest congestion.
- Ginger (1 teaspoon, grated): Helps loosen mucus and soothe a sore throat, making it an ideal ingredient for respiratory relief.
- Lemon (1 tablespoon, juice): Rich in vitamin C, lemon helps support the immune system and adds a refreshing, tangy flavor.
- Honey (1 tablespoon): A soothing agent that can calm throat irritation and also has mild antibacterial properties.
- Cinnamon (1/4 teaspoon): Known for its anti-inflammatory and antioxidant properties, it helps ease congestion.

Instructions:

1. Boil 2 cups of water in a saucepan.
2. Add basil leaves, grated ginger, and cinnamon. Let simmer for about 10 minutes.
3. Strain the brew into a cup.
4. Stir in honey and lemon juice. Adjust sweetness as needed.
- Drink 1-2 times a day to support respiratory health and clear chest congestion.
- Best consumed fresh, but can be stored in the fridge for up to 24 hours. Simply reheat before consuming.

Soothing Relief Balm

This balm is perfect for soothing sore muscles, dry skin, or any discomfort that requires a natural remedy. Combining the calming properties of essential oils and natural butters, it provides a gentle, nourishing treatment for areas of irritation.

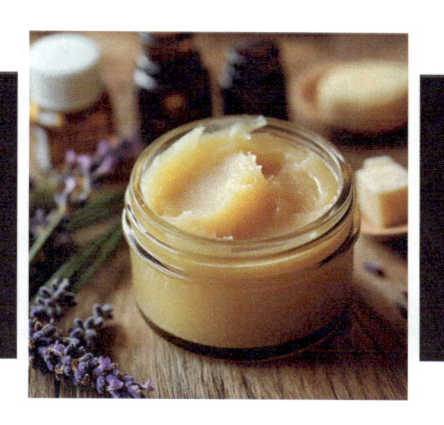

Ingredients:

- Coconut Oil (1/4 cup): A deeply moisturizing oil that softens skin and helps reduce inflammation.
- Beeswax (2 tablespoons): Acts as a natural emulsifier and provides a protective barrier for the skin, locking in moisture.
- Lavender Essential Oil (10 drops): Known for its soothing and anti-inflammatory properties, it helps calm irritated skin and relax the muscles.
- Peppermint Essential Oil (5 drops): Provides a cooling sensation, relieving muscle tension and inflammation.
- Eucalyptus Essential Oil (5 drops): Offers a refreshing effect that helps clear airways.
- Shea Butter (2 tablespoons): Nourishes and hydrates the skin, promoting healing.

Instructions:

1. In a double boiler, melt the beeswax and coconut oil together.
2. Once melted, remove from heat and stir in the shea butter until fully incorporated.
3. Add the essential oils and mix well.
4. Pour the mixture into a small glass jar or tin and let it cool completely before use.
- Gently apply a small amount of the balm to the affected area and massage in until absorbed. Reapply as needed.
- Keep in a cool, dry place. This balm can last for several months if stored properly.

Allergy-Ease Herbal Tea

This herbal tea blend is designed to naturally ease allergy symptoms by soothing inflammation and promoting a healthy immune response. It combines herbs traditionally used for their ability to relieve congestion, reduce histamine levels, and calm irritated airways.

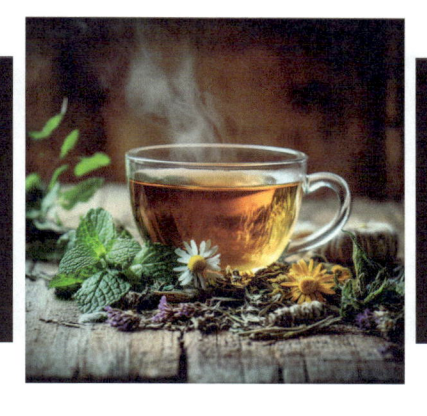

Ingredients:

- Nettle Leaf (1 teaspoon): Known for its anti-inflammatory properties, it helps reduce the symptoms of seasonal allergies.
- Peppermint Leaf (1 teaspoon): Offers a cooling sensation and helps open up airways, making breathing easier.
- Chamomile Flowers (1 teaspoon): Known for its calming effects, chamomile also helps reduce inflammation in the nasal passages.
- Lemon Balm (1 teaspoon): A mild sedative that can help soothe irritated tissues and calm the immune response.
- Echinacea Root (1/2 teaspoon): Supports the immune system and helps reduce the severity of allergic reactions.

Instructions:

1. Boil 2 cups of water.
2. Add all the herbs to a tea infuser or directly into the water.
3. Let steep for 10–15 minutes, then strain if necessary.
4. Sweeten with honey or stevia if desired.
- Enjoy 1–2 cups a day, especially during allergy season, to help ease symptoms and support the immune system.
- Store dried herbs in a cool, dry place. This tea blend can be made in larger batches and kept in an airtight container for up to 6 months.

Nettle Hay Fever Tincture

This tincture harnesses the power of nettle, a herb traditionally used to ease hay fever symptoms by reducing histamine production and inflammation. It's a natural remedy to help soothe the discomfort associated with seasonal allergies, offering a more gentle, herbal approach to managing hay fever.

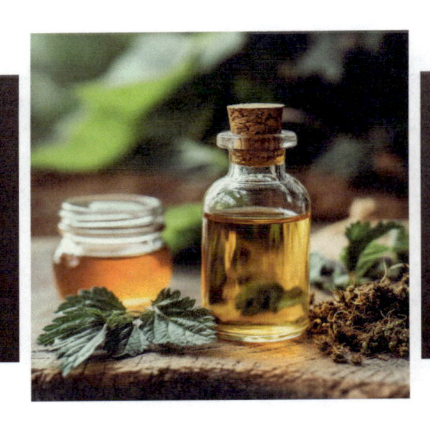

Ingredients:

- Nettle Leaf (2 tablespoons, dried): Acts as a natural antihistamine to reduce hay fever symptoms and support the respiratory system.
- Filtered Water (1/2 cup): Used as a base for extraction.
- Apple Cider Vinegar (1/2 cup): Extracts the active compounds from nettle and preserves the tincture.

Instructions:

1. Combine the dried nettle and apple cider vinegar in a glass jar.
2. Add water to cover the nettle, ensuring all ingredients are submerged.
3. Seal tightly and let sit in a cool, dark place for 2-3 weeks, shaking daily.
4. Strain and transfer to a dropper bottle.
- Take 1-2 droppers full (about 1/2-1 teaspoon) up to 3 times a day. It's best taken at the first sign of hay fever symptoms to manage reactions more effectively.
- Store in a cool, dark place. The tincture should last for 1-2 years when properly stored.

Mullein Mucus Buster

Mullein has long been used in herbal medicine to support respiratory health and alleviate congestion. This simple herbal remedy combines mullein with other helpful ingredients to create a soothing, mucus-clearing syrup designed to ease respiratory discomfort from colds, coughs, and bronchial issues.

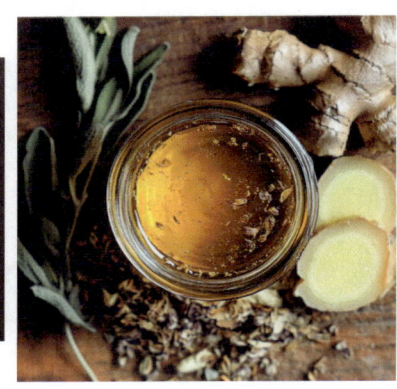

Ingredients:

- Mullein Leaf (1/2 cup dried): Known for its ability to help clear mucus from the lungs and soothe the respiratory tract.
- Licorice Root (1/4 cup dried): Supports lung health and helps soothe coughs while acting as an expectorant to loosen mucus.
- Honey (1/2 cup): Natural antibacterial and soothing agent that helps coat the throat, providing relief from irritation.
- Water (2 cups): Used to create the herbal infusion.
- Ginger Root (1 tablespoon, grated): Known for its anti-inflammatory properties and ability to support healthy digestion and respiratory function.

Instructions:

1. In a saucepan, bring 2 cups of water to a boil.
2. Add the mullein leaf, licorice root, and grated ginger to the boiling water.
3. Reduce heat and let simmer for 20-30 minutes.
4. Strain the herbs from the liquid and discard the solids.
5. Allow the liquid to cool slightly, then stir in the honey until it dissolves completely.
6. Pour the syrup into a glass jar or bottle for storage.
- Take 1 tablespoon of the syrup up to 3 times a day to help clear mucus and support respiratory health. Store the syrup in a cool, dark place for up to 2 weeks,

Onion Heat Relief Wrap

Onions have long been used in traditional remedies for their soothing and anti-inflammatory properties. This heat relief wrap combines onions with natural ingredients to create a therapeutic treatment for muscle aches, tension, or even chest congestion.

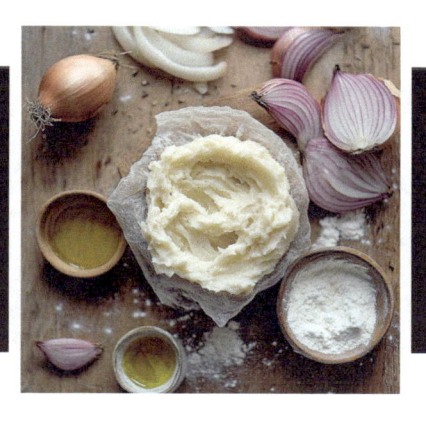

Ingredients:

- Onion (1 large): Contains sulfur compounds known for their anti-inflammatory and analgesic effects, helping to relieve muscle pain or congestion.
- Olive Oil (2 tablespoons): Moisturizes the skin while providing a smooth base for the wrap.
- Flour (1 tablespoon): Helps create a paste-like consistency to hold the onions in place when applied.
- Cheesecloth or Soft Cloth (for wrapping): To wrap the mixture securely on the affected area.

Instructions:

- Slice the onion into thin rings and place in a bowl. Then heat olive oil in a small pan, then sauté the onion slices until they become soft and release their juices.
- Once the onions have softened, remove them from the heat and mix in the flour to form a paste-like consistency.
- Place the onion paste onto a piece of soft cloth.
- Wrap the cloth around the affected area (such as the chest, back, or joints) to create a compress.
- Secure the wrap in place and allow it to sit for 20-30 minutes, then remove and discard the onion paste.
- Apply the wrap to sore muscles, joints, or congested areas to help relieve pain and discomfort. Repeat up to 2-3 times a day.

Cool Down Vinegar Wraps

Vinegar wraps are a natural remedy used to reduce inflammation, cool the body, and soothe irritated skin. This simple treatment is perfect for hot, swollen areas or even to ease a fever.

Ingredients:

- Apple Cider Vinegar (1/2 cup): Known for its cooling and soothing properties, apple cider vinegar helps reduce inflammation and can balance the skin's pH.
- Cold Water (1/2 cup): Helps dilute the vinegar and enhance the cooling effect.
- Cloth or Cheesecloth (for wrapping): Used to apply the vinegar solution evenly and securely on the skin.

Instructions:

1. Mix apple cider vinegar and cold water in a bowl.
2. Soak a cloth or cheesecloth in the mixture, ensuring it's fully saturated.
3. Wring out any excess liquid to avoid dripping.
4. Place the damp cloth on the affected area (e.g., a sunburn, sore muscles, or irritated skin).
5. Leave the wrap on for 15–20 minutes, then remove and discard.
- Apply the wrap to inflamed or heated areas, such as a feverish forehead, swollen joints, or sunburns. You can repeat this 2–3 times a day, as needed.
- Use the vinegar mixture fresh or store it in the fridge for up to 2 days.

Anti-Fever Elixir

This soothing elixir is designed to help reduce fever, promote sweating to regulate body temperature, and relieve discomfort during illness. It combines natural ingredients that have cooling and calming effects, helping to alleviate fever symptoms.

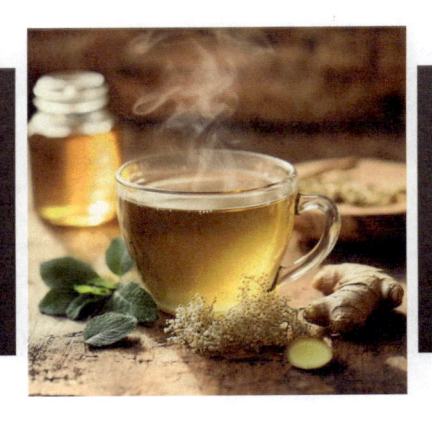

Ingredients:

- Elderflower (1 tablespoon): Known for its ability to promote sweating, elderflower helps lower body temperature naturally.a
- Lemon Balm (1 teaspoon): Offers a calming effect and supports the body's ability to regulate fever.
- Ginger Root (1/2 teaspoon): A warming herb that stimulates circulation and helps reduce fever.
- Honey (1 teaspoon): Soothes the throat and adds natural sweetness.
- Apple Cider Vinegar (1 tablespoon): A natural remedy to help balance the body's pH and assist in lowering a fever.

Instructions:

1. Boil 1 cup of water and pour it over elderflower and lemon balm.
2. Let the herbs steep for 5-10 minutes, then strain.
3. Add ginger, honey, and apple cider vinegar to the herbal infusion.
4. Stir well until the ingredients are fully blended.
- Drink this elixir 2–3 times a day to help manage fever and promote healing. Be sure to stay hydrated while using this remedy.
- Best when consumed fresh. If you have leftovers, store in the fridge for up to 24 hours.

Herbal Fever Compress

A simple herbal fever compress to help ease discomfort and regulate body temperature during a fever. This remedy uses a few soothing ingredients to provide relief without overwhelming your system.

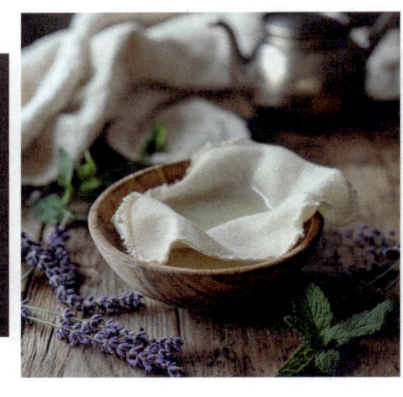

Ingredients:

- Peppermint (2 teaspoons): Naturally cooling and helps relieve fever-related headaches and discomfort.
- Lavender (1 teaspoon): Known for its calming properties, it soothes and helps reduce stress caused by fevers.
- Warm Water (1 cup): To steep the herbs and create a soothing compress.

Instructions:

1. Boil 1 cup of water and pour it over the peppermint and lavender.
2. Let the herbs steep for 5–10 minutes.
3. Strain out the herbs and allow the liquid to cool slightly.
4. Soak a clean cloth in the herbal water, then wring it out to remove excess liquid.
5. Apply the cloth to the forehead, neck, or other feverish areas. Keep it on for 10–20 minutes, re-soaking if necessary.
- Use the compress as needed, especially on the forehead or neck, to relieve fever and cool the body down.
- Any remaining herbal liquid can be stored in the fridge for up to 24 hours.

Snore Relief Jelly

This soothing jelly is designed to help ease snoring by promoting relaxation of the respiratory muscles and reducing nasal congestion. Using natural ingredients that support healthy airflow, this remedy is perfect for those seeking a restful night's sleep.

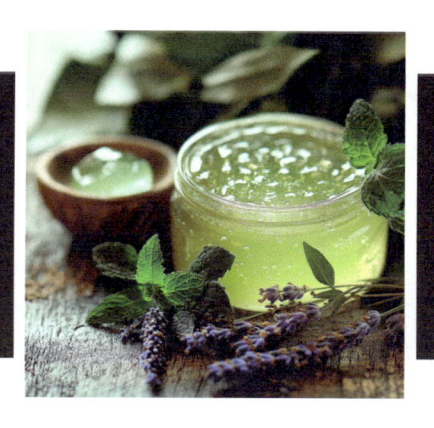

Ingredients:

- Peppermint Oil (5 drops): Known for its cooling properties, peppermint oil helps open up airways and can relieve nasal congestion.
- Eucalyptus Oil (5 drops): Eucalyptus is known for its ability to clear nasal passages, making it easier to breathe through the night.
- Honey (1 tablespoon): A soothing agent for the throat and helps to calm the airways.
- Aloe Vera Gel (2 tablespoons): Provides a cooling effect, reducing irritation in the throat and nasal passages.
- Lavender Oil (3 drops): Promotes relaxation and improves sleep quality, which can help reduce snoring.

Instructions:

1. In a small bowl, mix aloe vera gel and honey until smooth.
2. Add peppermint, eucalyptus, and lavender oils to the mixture.
3. Stir well until everything is fully blended.

- Before bed, apply a small amount of the Snore Relief Jelly to the chest, throat, and around the nose to help ease snoring. Reapply if necessary during the night.
- Store the jelly in an airtight container in the refrigerator for up to 1 week.

Turmeric Tonic for Inflammation

This soothing tonic combines the powerful anti-inflammatory benefits of turmeric with other natural ingredients to help reduce inflammation and support overall joint health. Perfect for those seeking a natural remedy to soothe sore muscles or joint discomfort.

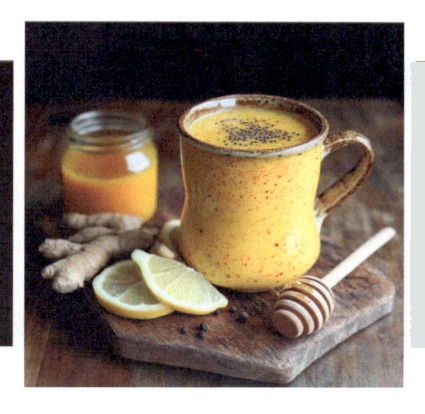

Ingredients:

- Turmeric Powder (1 teaspoon): Contains curcumin, a compound with potent anti-inflammatory properties that can help reduce pain and swelling.
- Ginger (1/2 teaspoon, grated or powdered): Known for its ability to fight inflammation and improve circulation, ginger also enhances the effectiveness of turmeric.
- Honey (1 tablespoon): Soothes the throat and acts as a natural anti-inflammatory, promoting overall healing.
- Lemon Juice (1 tablespoon): Adds a refreshing tang while aiding digestion and detoxifying the body.
- Black Pepper (a pinch): Contains piperine, which enhances the absorption of curcumin, making turmeric more effective.

Instructions:

1. In a mug, combine turmeric, ginger, honey, and lemon juice.
2. Add a pinch of black pepper and mix well.
3. Pour in hot water (about 1 cup) and stir until the honey is dissolved.

- Drink 1-2 times a day, especially during flare-ups of inflammation, or as part of your daily routine for general wellness.
- Best consumed fresh. If needed, store the mixture in a sealed container in the refrigerator for up to 2 days.

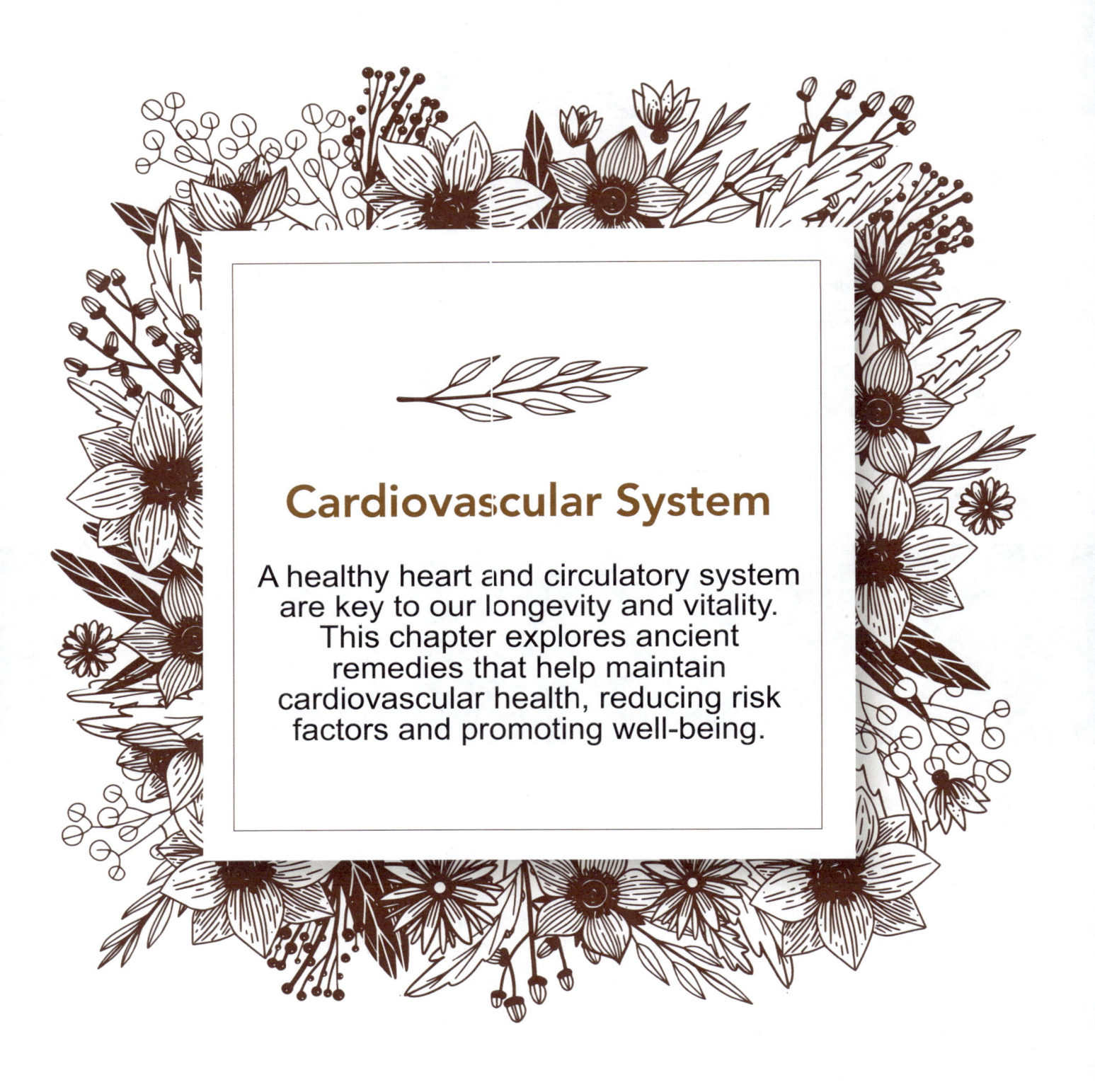

Cardiovascular System

A healthy heart and circulatory system are key to our longevity and vitality. This chapter explores ancient remedies that help maintain cardiovascular health, reducing risk factors and promoting well-being.

Arterial De-Clogger

This potent herbal remedy is designed to support arterial health by promoting circulation and reducing plaque build-up. The herbs in this formulation are believed to help strengthen blood vessels, improve flow, and cleanse the circulatory system.

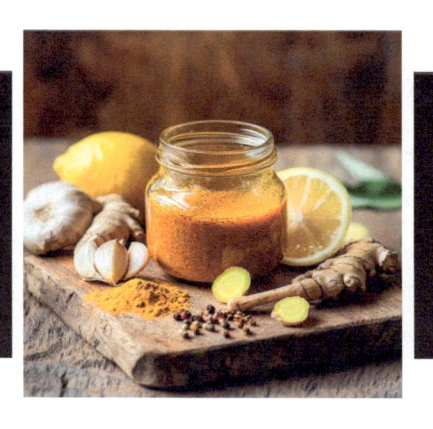

Ingredients:

- Garlic (2-3 cloves): Supports cholesterol and blood pressure.
- Turmeric (1 tsp): Reduces plaque with anti-inflammatory properties.
- Ginger (1 tsp): Improves circulation and reduces clotting.
- Cayenne (1/4 tsp): Boosts blood flow and clears blockages.
- Apple Cider Vinegar (1 tbsp): Detoxifies and regulates cholesterol.
- Lemon (juice of 1): Supports arterial health and detox.
- Honey (1 tbsp): Adds antioxidants and supports heart health.

Instructions:

1. In a jar, combine the garlic, turmeric, ginger, cayenne pepper, and lemon juice.
2. Pour in the apple cider vinegar and stir well.
3. Add honey for taste and additional health benefits.
4. Let the mixture sit for about 24 hours in a cool, dark place, then strain.
- Store in an airtight jar in the refrigerator.
- Take 1 tablespoon of the mixture daily, preferably in the morning on an empty stomach, to help cleanse the arteries and improve circulation.
- Keep refrigerated for up to 2 weeks.

Warming Turmeric and Cayenne Balm to Promote Circulation

This warming balm combines the powerful anti-inflammatory and circulation-boosting properties of turmeric and cayenne pepper. It can be used to relieve muscle aches, stiffness, and improve blood flow to the targeted areas.

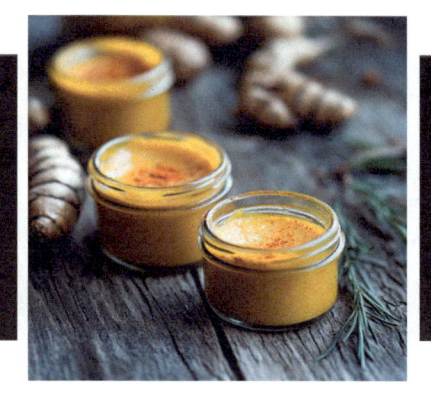

Ingredients:

- Turmeric Powder (1 tablespoon): Known for its anti-inflammatory and pain-relieving properties, turmeric helps reduce muscle soreness and improve circulation.
- Cayenne Pepper (1/2 teaspoon): Contains capsaicin, which stimulates blood flow and can help relieve pain and improve circulation.
- Beeswax (2 tablespoons): Creates a solid base for the balm and helps lock in moisture.
- Coconut Oil (1/4 cup): Acts as a carrier oil and provides hydration while promoting circulation.
- Olive Oil (1/4 cup): Adds to the moisturizing and healing properties of the balm.

Instructions:

1. In a double boiler, melt the beeswax, coconut oil, and olive oil together.
2. Once melted, stir in the turmeric powder and cayenne pepper. Mix well.
3. Pour the balm into small jars or tins and let it set at room temperature.
4. Optional: You can add a few drops of lavender or peppermint essential oil for additional soothing effects.
- Massage a small amount of balm onto sore muscles or areas where you want to promote circulation.
- Keep in a cool, dry place for up to 6 months.

Cinnamon Infusion for Blood Pressure

This simple yet powerful cinnamon infusion can help support healthy blood pressure levels. Cinnamon is widely known for its potential to improve circulation, lower blood sugar, and support heart health, making it a great addition to any wellness routine.

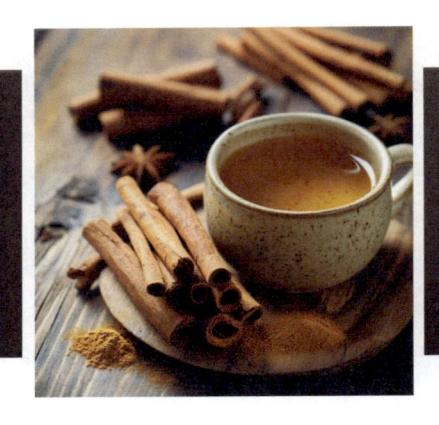

Ingredients:

- Cinnamon Sticks (1-2 sticks): Known for its ability to improve circulation and help regulate blood pressure.
- Water (2 cups): The base for your infusion.
- Honey (1 teaspoon, optional): Adds natural sweetness and may have mild blood pressure-lowering effects.

Instructions:

1. Boil 2 cups of water in a small saucepan.
2. Add 1-2 cinnamon sticks and reduce the heat to a simmer.
3. Let the cinnamon steep in the water for about 10-15 minutes.
4. Strain the liquid into a mug, add honey if desired, and enjoy.
- Drink 1-2 cups per day, ideally in the morning or evening, as part of a balanced lifestyle to help maintain healthy blood pressure.
- The cinnamon infusion is best enjoyed fresh. However, you can refrigerate any leftover liquid for up to 24 hours and reheat it when needed.

Heart Harmony Elixir with Hawthorn Berry

This Heart Harmony Elixir combines hawthorn berry with other heart-healthy herbs to create a soothing and supportive blend for heart health. Hawthorn berries have long been celebrated for their ability to strengthen the cardiovascular system, improve circulation, and support overall heart function.

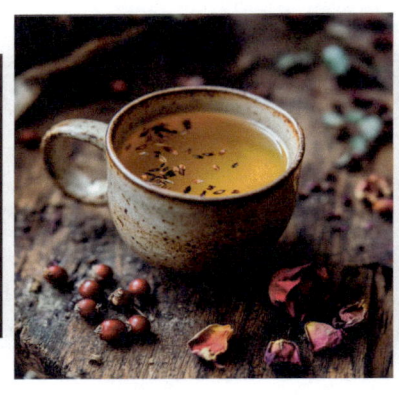

Ingredients:

- Hawthorn Berry (1 tablespoon, dried): Known for its ability to support heart health by improving circulation and reducing blood pressure.
- Rose Petals (1 tablespoon, dried): Used for their calming and anti-inflammatory effects, promoting overall cardiovascular wellness.
- Lemon Balm (1 teaspoon, dried): Known to relax the heart and relieve stress
- Raw Honey (1 teaspoon, optional): Adds natural sweetness and supports overall health with its antibacterial and anti-inflammatory properties.
- Water (2 cups): Acts as the base for your infusion.

Instructions:

1. Boil 2 cups of water in a saucepan.
2. Add 1 tablespoon of dried hawthorn berries, 1 tablespoon of rose petals, and 1 teaspoon of lemon balm to the water.
3. Reduce the heat and let the mixture simmer for about 15 minutes.
4. Strain the liquid into a mug and add honey if desired.
- Drink 1 cup per day, especially during moments of stress or after physical activity, to promote heart health and relaxation.
- Best consumed fresh, but can be stored in the refrigerator for up to 24 hours. Reheat before drinking.

Garlic and Lemon Tonic for Cholesterol Management

This Garlic and Lemon Tonic is a natural remedy that can help support cholesterol management and cardiovascular health. Both garlic and lemon are known for their beneficial effects on the heart, and when combined, they create a simple, yet potent tonic.

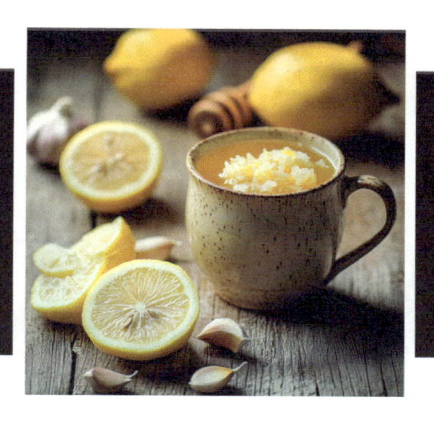

Ingredients:

- Garlic (2 cloves, minced): Garlic is rich in allicin, which helps lower cholesterol levels and prevent plaque buildup in arteries. It can also improve circulation and reduce blood pressure.
- Lemon (1, juiced): Lemons are high in vitamin C and antioxidants that support healthy cholesterol levels and reduce inflammation, which is vital for overall heart health.
- Raw Honey (optional, 1 teaspoon): Honey has antibacterial properties and can also help soothe the throat and improve the taste of the tonic.
- Water (1 cup): Water serves as the base for the tonic, helping to hydrate and dissolve the ingredients.

Instructions:

1. Mince the garlic cloves and juice the lemon.
2. In a small saucepan, bring 1 cup of water to a boil and add the minced garlic and let it simmer for 5–10 minutes to extract its beneficial compounds.
3. Remove from heat, add the lemon juice and honey (if using), then stir well.
4. Strain the mixture into a cup and enjoy while warm.

- Consume this tonic once a day, preferably in the morning, to help manage cholesterol levels and promote overall cardiovascular health.
- Best enjoyed fresh, but can be stored in the fridge for up to 24 hours. Reheat gently before drinking.

Hibiscus Tea for Cardiovascular Support

Hibiscus tea is a well-known herbal remedy with a range of health benefits, particularly for cardiovascular health. Rich in antioxidants and anthocyanins, hibiscus has been shown to help lower blood pressure, support cholesterol levels, and enhance overall heart health.

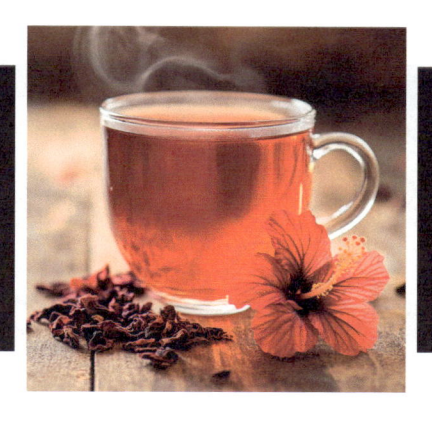

Ingredients:

- Dried hibiscus flowers (1-2 teaspoons): Known for their high content of antioxidants and anthocyanins that support heart health.
- Water (1 cup): For brewing the tea.
- Optional sweetener (honey or stevia): To taste, if you prefer a sweeter tea.

Instructions:

1. Boil 1 cup of water in a kettle or saucepan.
2. Add the dried hibiscus flowers to a teapot or mug.
3. Pour the hot water over the flowers and let it steep for 5-10 minutes, depending on your preferred strength.
4. Strain the tea into a cup and sweeten with honey or stevia if desired.
5. Enjoy the tea warm or chilled as a refreshing drink throughout the day.

- Enjoy a cup of hibiscus tea daily to support cardiovascular health and maintain a balanced blood pressure level.
- Store unused dried hibiscus flowers in a cool, dry place, away from direct sunlight, to preserve their potency for up to a year.

Beetroot and Aronia Juice for Circulatory Health

This potent juice combines the powerful properties of beetroot and aronia berries to support circulatory health. Both ingredients are rich in antioxidants and compounds known to help improve blood circulation, lower blood pressure, and protect the cardiovascular system.

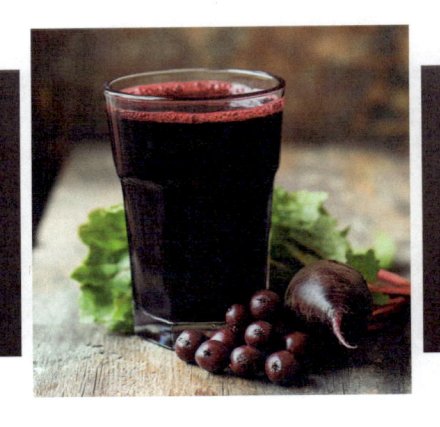

Ingredients:

- Fresh beetroot (1 medium-sized root): Contains nitrates, which may help improve blood flow and lower blood pressure.
- Aronia berries (1/4 cup): High in anthocyanins, which have antioxidant and anti-inflammatory effects that benefit heart health.
- Water or coconut water (1 cup): To help blend the ingredients smoothly.
- Optional sweetener (honey or stevia): If you prefer a sweeter taste.

Instructions:

1. Peel and chop the beetroot into small pieces.
2. Place the beetroot and aronia berries into a blender or juicer.
3. Add water or coconut water to help blend the mixture.
4. Blend until smooth, strain for a thinner juice.
5. Sweeten to taste with honey if desired.
6. Pour into a glass and enjoy.

- Drink 1/2 to 1 cup daily to support healthy circulation and cardiovascular function. For best results, consume regularly as part of a heart-healthy lifestyle.
- Store any leftover juice in the refrigerator for up to 2 days.

Blood Vessel Care with Butcher's Broom

Butcher's broom is a traditional herb used to promote healthy circulation and support blood vessel function. It is particularly beneficial for conditions related to poor circulation, such as varicose veins, hemorrhoids, and general vascular health. The active compounds in butcher's broom, help constrict blood vessels and improve blood flow, which can reduce swelling and alleviate discomfort associated with circulatory issues.

Ingredients:

- Dried butcher's broom root (1 teaspoon): Contains ruscogenins, which improve circulation and help with venous health.
- Water (1 cup): To steep the herb.
- Optional sweetener (honey): For added taste if desired.

Instructions:

1. Boil 1 cup of water in a saucepan.
2. Add 1 teaspoon of dried butcher's broom root to the water.
3. Let it steep for 10–15 minutes.
4. Strain out the herb and pour the liquid into a mug.
5. Optional: Add honey to taste for a sweeter flavor.

- Consume one cup of this herbal infusion daily to support blood vessel health and circulation. It can be used regularly, especially if you're prone to circulatory issues.
- Store any leftover infusion in the refrigerator and consume within 24 hours.

Bilberry Heart Drops

Bilberries are known for their potent antioxidant content and their ability to support cardiovascular health. They contain anthocyanins, compounds that help improve blood flow, reduce inflammation, and strengthen the blood vessels. These heart-supportive properties make bilberry an ideal herb for promoting overall cardiovascular health and protecting the heart from oxidative damage.

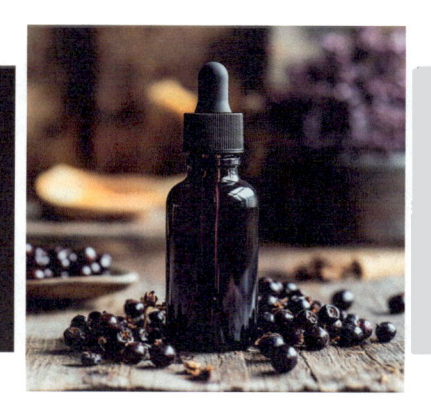

Ingredients:

- Bilberry (1 tablespoon, dried): Promotes heart health and supports circulation due to its high levels of anthocyanins.
- Filtered Water (1/2 cup): Used as a base for infusion.
- Apple Cider Vinegar (1/2 cup): Extracts the active compounds in bilberry and aids heart health.

Instructions:

1. Combine the dried bilberry and apple cider vinegar in a glass jar.
2. Add water to cover the bilberry completely.
3. Seal tightly and let sit in a cool, dark place for 2-3 weeks, shaking daily.
4. Strain and transfer to a dropper bottle.
- Take 1-2 droppers full (approximately 30-60 drops) of bilberry tincture in water or juice 1-2 times per day to support heart health and improve circulation.
- Store the tincture in a cool, dark place and use within 6-12 months.

Horse Chestnut Cooling Gel for Varicose Veins

Horse chestnut (Aesculus hippocastanum) is a well-known herbal remedy for varicose veins due to its ability to strengthen blood vessels and improve circulation. This cooling gel combines the soothing properties of horse chestnut with natural ingredients that help alleviate swelling and discomfort associated with varicose veins.

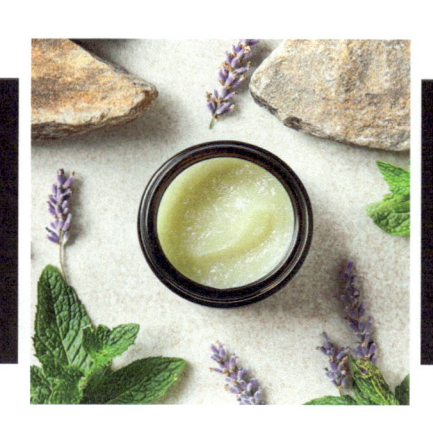

Ingredients:

- Horse Chestnut extract (2 tablespoons): Contains aescin, which helps reduce swelling and improves blood flow.
- Aloe Vera gel (1/4 cup): Soothes and cools the skin, reducing inflammation.
- Peppermint essential oil (5 drops): Provides a cooling effect and relieves pain.
- Lavender essential oil (3 drops): Calms the skin and has anti-inflammatory properties.
- Carrier oil (such as jojoba or sweet almond oil, 1 tablespoon): Used to help blend the ingredients together.

Instructions:

1. In a small bowl, mix the horse chestnut extract with the aloe vera gel and carrier oil.
2. Add the peppermint and lavender essential oils and stir well to combine.
3. Pour the mixture into a sterilized container with a tight-fitting lid.
4. Store the gel in the fridge for added cooling effect.
- Apply the gel to the affected area (e.g., over varicose veins) 2-3 times daily. Massage gently into the skin, using upward strokes.
- Keep the gel in a cool place (preferably refrigerated) and use within 2-3 weeks.

Young Heart Elixir

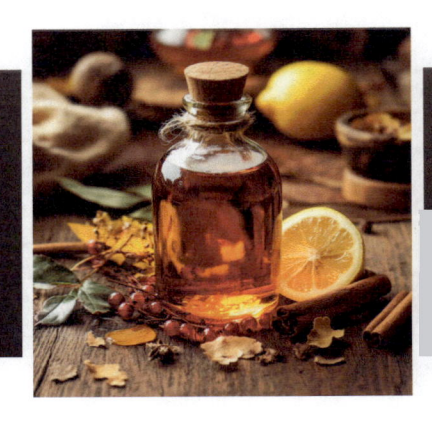

This heart-supporting elixir is crafted with nourishing herbs and ingredients that help maintain cardiovascular health and promote vitality. The blend of antioxidant-rich botanicals helps support circulation, strengthen the heart, and improve overall heart function.

Ingredients:

- Hawthorn Berry (1 tbsp): Improves circulation and strengthens the heart.
- Rose Petals (1 tbsp): Supports heart health and reduces stress.
- Ginkgo Biloba (1 tsp): Promotes blood flow and energy.
- Cinnamon (1/2 tsp): Improves circulation and regulates blood sugar.
- Honey (1 tbsp): Anti-inflammatory and immune-boosting.
- Apple Cider Vinegar (1 tbsp): Supports circulation and detoxifies.
- Lemon (juice of 1 lemon): Supports arterial health and detox.

Instructions:

1. Steep hawthorn, rose petals, and ginkgo in 1 cup hot water for 10-15 minutes.
2. Strain, then stir in honey, vinegar, cinnamon, and lemon juice.
3. Let cool to room temperature and store in the fridge.

- Take 1 tablespoon daily for heart health and circulation.
- Refrigerate for up to two weeks.

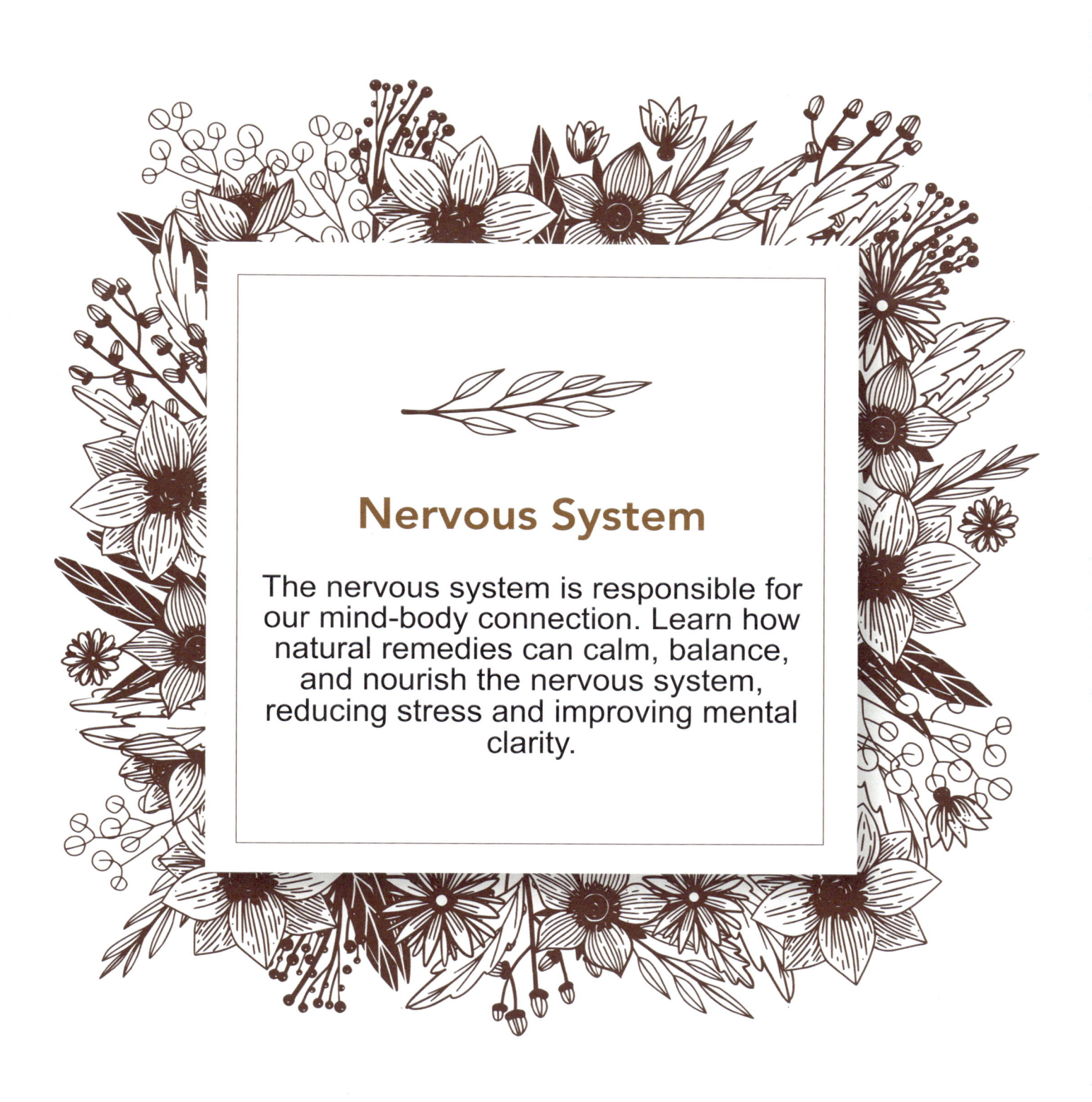

Nervous System

The nervous system is responsible for our mind-body connection. Learn how natural remedies can calm, balance, and nourish the nervous system, reducing stress and improving mental clarity.

Memory Elixir

This Memory Elixir is a blend of herbs and ingredients traditionally known to enhance cognitive function, improve focus, and support mental clarity. Ideal for those looking to boost memory retention and concentration naturally.

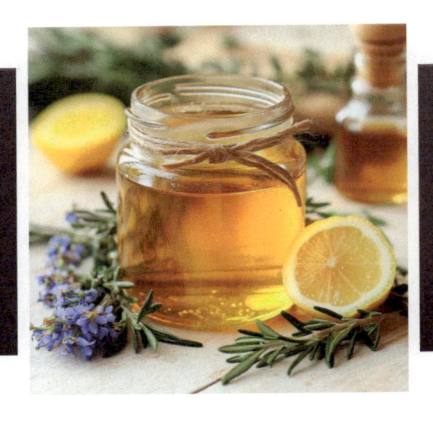

Ingredients:

- Rosemary (1 teaspoon, dried): Known for its ability to improve memory and stimulate mental clarity.
- Ginkgo Biloba (1 teaspoon, dried): Supports brain health and circulation, improving cognitive function.
- Bacopa Monnieri (1 teaspoon, dried): An herb traditionally used to enhance memory and reduce anxiety, known for its cognitive-boosting properties.
- Lemon Balm (1 teaspoon, dried): Helps reduce stress and anxiety
- Honey (1 tablespoon): Adds sweetness and acts as a natural anti-inflammatory, while also supporting immune health.
- Lemon Juice (1 tablespoon): Provides vitamin C and antioxidants that support overall brain health.

Instructions:

- Combine all herbs in a heat-safe container.
- Pour 1 cup of hot water over the herbs and let it steep for about 5-7 minutes.
- Strain the herbs and pour the elixir into a glass.
- Stir in honey and lemon juice for added flavor and benefits.
- Drink 1-2 times a day to support cognitive function, enhance memory, and improve focus.
- Store any leftover elixir in the refrigerator for up to 24 hours.

Brain Boosting Tonic

This Brain Boosting Tonic combines natural herbs and ingredients traditionally used to support cognitive health, improve mental clarity, and enhance focus. It's ideal for those looking to sharpen their minds and support long-term brain function.

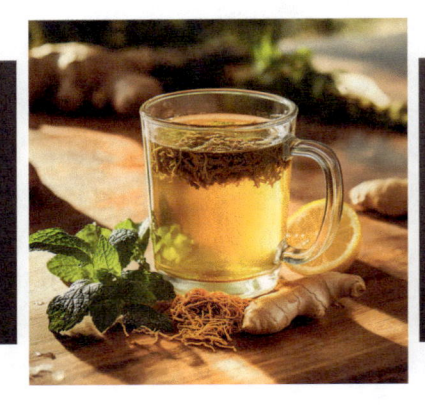

Ingredients:

- Ginseng (1 teaspoon, dried): Known for enhancing cognitive performance and reducing mental fatigue.
- Gotu Kola (1 teaspoon, dried): A powerful herb that supports brain health and improves memory and concentration.
- Peppermint (1 teaspoon, dried): Known to boost focus and mental clarity.
- Lemon Balm (1 teaspoon, dried): Helps reduce stress making it easier to concentrate.
- Honey (1 tablespoon): A natural sweetener that supports overall well-being and provides an energy boost.
- Ginger (1/2 teaspoon, dried or fresh): Known for stimulating circulation and improving brain function.

Instructions:

1. Combine all the dried herbs in a heat-safe container.
2. Pour 1 cup of boiling water over the herbs.
3. Let it steep for about 5-7 minutes, then strain the herbs out.
4. Stir in honey for sweetness and a boost of nutrients.
- Drink 1 cup of this Brain Boosting Tonic once or twice daily to support brain health, mental clarity, and focus.
- Store any leftover tonic in the refrigerator for up to 24 hours.

Natural Brain Booster

This powerful blend of herbs and natural ingredients is designed to enhance cognitive function, improve memory, and support mental clarity. Perfect for a natural pick-me-up when you need to stay sharp throughout the day.

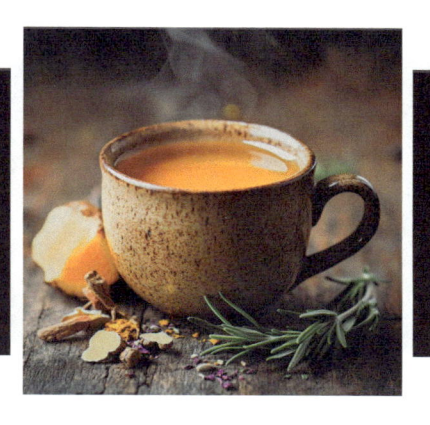

Ingredients:

- Ginkgo Biloba (1 teaspoon, dried): Traditionally used to improve memory, focus, and overall cognitive function.
- Rosemary (1 teaspoon, dried): Known for enhancing memory and concentration by improving blood circulation to the brain.
- Turmeric (1/4 teaspoon, ground): Contains curcumin, which supports brain health and reduces inflammation, contributing to overall cognitive health.
- Lemon Balm (1 teaspoon, dried): Helps to alleviate stress, improve mood, and boost mental clarity.
- Honey (1 tablespoon): Naturally sweetens the tonic while providing an additional energy boost.

Instructions:

1. Combine all dried herbs in a heat-safe mug or teapot.
2. Pour boiling water over the herbs and steep for 5-7 minutes.
3. Strain out the herbs, then stir in honey.
4. Drink while hot for a refreshing and energizing experience.
- Consume 1 cup daily to enhance brain function, improve focus, and support memory.
- Store any leftover tonic in the refrigerator for up to 24 hours.

Brain Power Mushroom Elixir

This elixir uses medicinal mushrooms to support cognitive function and mental clarity, without the need for extra ingredients. The reduced list of ingredients still provides powerful brain-boosting benefits.

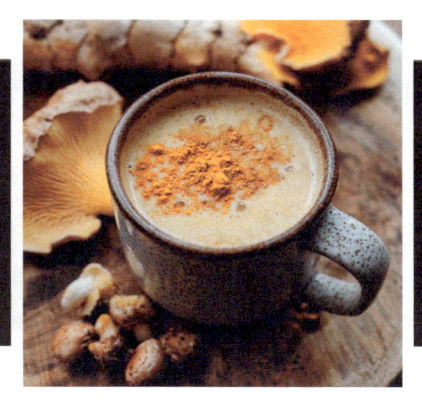

Ingredients:

- Lion's Mane Mushroom Powder (1 teaspoon): Known for enhancing cognitive function and nerve regeneration.
- Reishi Mushroom Powder (1 teaspoon): Helps reduce stress and supports brain health.
- Cordyceps Mushroom Powder (1/2 teaspoon): Increases energy levels and mental focus.
- Turmeric (1/4 teaspoon, ground): Contains curcumin, known for its anti-inflammatory effects on the brain.
- Coconut Milk (1/2 cup): A creamy base for hydration and providing healthy fats for brain function.

Instructions:

1. In a small saucepan, combine coconut milk, Lion's Mane, Reishi, Cordyceps, and turmeric.
2. Heat gently over medium heat, stirring occasionally until warm (not boiling).
3. Pour into a mug and enjoy.

- Drink 1 cup daily to support mental clarity and cognitive health.
- Best consumed fresh but can be stored in the refrigerator for up to 24 hours.

Mind Sharpening Infusion

This infusion blends herbs traditionally used to support mental clarity, focus, and cognitive function, creating a refreshing drink that promotes alertness and concentration.

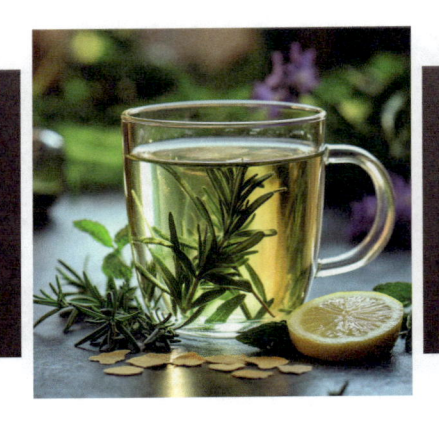

Ingredients:

- Ginkgo Biloba (1 teaspoon): Known for improving memory and cognitive function by increasing blood flow to the brain.
- Rosemary (1/2 teaspoon): Helps with mental clarity and has been shown to improve concentration and memory.
- Lemon Balm (1 teaspoon): Provides calming effects while enhancing focus and concentration.
- Peppermint (1/2 teaspoon): Stimulates the mind and helps reduce mental fatigue.
- Green Tea (1 bag or 1 teaspoon): Provides gentle caffeine for sustained energy and alertness, supporting overall brain function.

Instructions:

1. Boil 2 cups of water in a kettle or saucepan.
2. Add all herbs (or a tea bag of green tea) and let steep for 5–7 minutes.
3. Strain the herbs if necessary, and pour the infusion into a mug.
4. Enjoy the infusion as is, or add a little honey or lemon for flavor.

- Drink 1–2 times per day to support mental sharpness, especially during long work sessions or study periods.
- Best consumed fresh, but can be refrigerated for up to 24 hours if needed.

Ginkgo Biloba Focus Fuel

This energizing blend harnesses the power of Ginkgo Biloba to support mental clarity, concentration, and memory. Known for its ability to improve blood circulation to the brain, this infusion can help boost cognitive function, making it an excellent choice when you need focus and sharpness throughout the day.

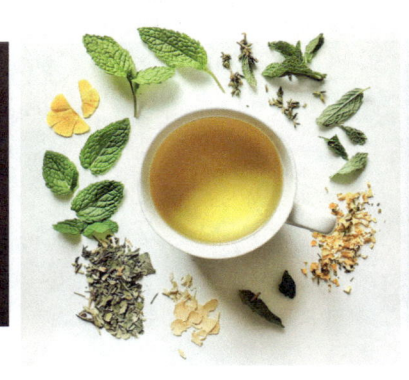

Ingredients:

- Ginkgo Biloba (1 teaspoon): A potent herb that enhances circulation to the brain, improving memory and cognitive performance.
- Green Tea (1 bag or 1 teaspoon): A gentle source of caffeine, providing steady energy without the jitters while boosting brain function.
- Lemon Balm (1 teaspoon): Offers calming properties while helping to focus the mind.
- Peppermint (1/2 teaspoon): Stimulates mental clarity and reduces mental fatigue.

Instructions:

1. Boil 2 cups of water.
2. Add all ingredients into the water and let it steep for 5–7 minutes.
3. Strain and pour into a mug.
4. Add honey or lemon if desired for extra flavor.

- Drink 1–2 times a day, especially before studying, working, or whenever you need to enhance mental clarity and focus.
- Consume fresh, or store in the fridge for up to 24 hours.

Anti-Migraine Syrup

This soothing syrup is formulated with herbs known for their ability to relieve headache pain and reduce migraine symptoms. The blend combines anti-inflammatory, analgesic, and calming ingredients that may help ease the intensity of a migraine and promote relaxation.

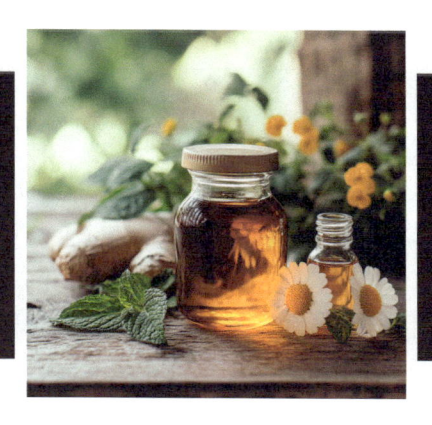

Ingredients:

- Feverfew (1 teaspoon): Widely used for migraine prevention and relief, this herb helps to reduce the frequency and severity of headaches.
- Ginger Root (1 teaspoon): Known for its anti-inflammatory properties, ginger helps to reduce pain and nausea associated with migraines.
- Peppermint Oil (3–5 drops): Provides a cooling sensation and can relieve tension headaches when applied topically or consumed.
- Lemon Balm (1 teaspoon): Calms the nervous system and helps to ease tension and stress, often triggers for migraines.
- Honey (1 tablespoon): Adds natural sweetness and helps with the absorption of the herbs while soothing the throat.

Instructions:

1. In a saucepan, combine 2 cups of water with all of the ingredients.
2. Bring to a gentle simmer for 10–15 minutes, allowing the herbs to infuse.
3. Strain the syrup into a clean glass jar or bottle.
4. Allow to cool and store in the fridge.
- Take 1 tablespoon every 3–4 hours during a migraine episode, or 1 tablespoon daily as a preventative measure.
- Store the syrup in the fridge for up to 1 week.

Herbal Blend for Headache Relief

This herbal blend is designed to relieve the pain and tension of headaches through a mix of soothing, anti-inflammatory, and muscle-relaxing ingredients. It's a simple and natural remedy to calm the nervous system and ease the discomfort caused by headaches.

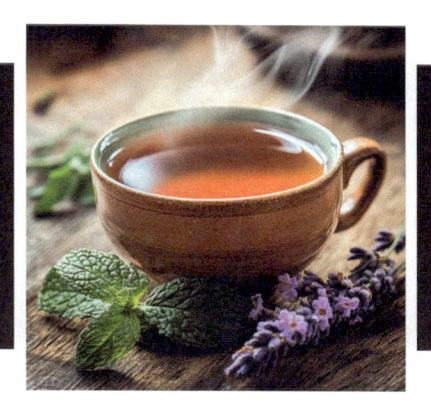

Ingredients:

- Lavender (1 teaspoon): helps reduce stress and tension, which can alleviate headache pain.
- Peppermint (1 teaspoon): Acts as a natural analgesic, peppermint oil helps soothe headaches, particularly tension headaches, by improving circulation and relieving muscle tightness.
- Ginger (1 teaspoon): This herb has anti-inflammatory properties that can help reduce headache symptoms and nausea that often accompanies migraines.
- Chamomile (1 teaspoon): Chamomile is gentle yet effective for its anti-inflammatory and calming properties.
- Lemon Balm (1 teaspoon): can help reduce anxiety and ease headaches brought on by stress or tension.

Instructions:

1. Boil 2 cups of water in a saucepan.
2. Add all of the herbs and allow them to steep for 10-15 minutes.
3. Strain the herbs from the water and pour the infusion into a mug.
4. Optional: Add honey for a touch of sweetness if desired.
5. Drink 1 cup of this herbal tea during a headache, or regularly to prevent headaches caused by stress or tension.
- Store any unused dried herbs in a cool, dry place, away from sunlight.

Moon Milk for Better Sleep

Moon Milk is a calming, herbal beverage that promotes relaxation and better sleep. This recipe combines traditional ingredients known for their ability to reduce stress and prepare the body for restful sleep.

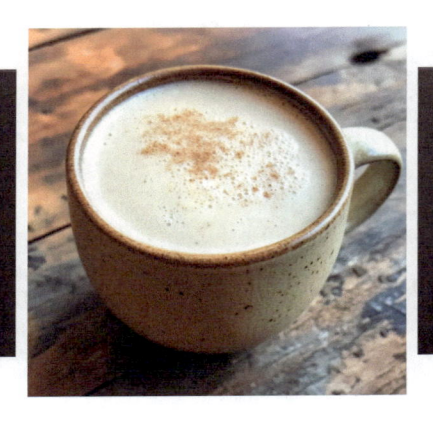

Ingredients:

- Turmeric (1/2 tsp): Known for its anti-inflammatory properties, turmeric also helps calm the nervous system, preparing the body for sleep.
- Ashwagandha (1/2 tsp): This adaptogen is celebrated for its stress-relieving properties and ability to improve sleep quality by regulating cortisol levels.
- Cinnamon (1/2 tsp):helps balance blood sugar levels and promotes relaxation.
- Ginger (1/4 tsp): calms discomfort and promotes a relaxed state conducive to sleep.
- Nutmeg (1/4 tsp): helps to calm the mind and support deep sleep.
- Warm Milk (1 cup): Traditionally used to enhance sleep due to its tryptophan content, which helps regulate sleep cycles.

Instructions:

1. Heat the milk in a saucepan until warm (but not boiling).
2. Add all the spices to the milk and stir gently to combine.
3. Let the mixture steep for 5-10 minutes.
4. Strain and pour into a cup. Add honey or maple syrup for sweetness if desired.
- Enjoy a cup of Moon Milk 30 minutes before bedtime to help calm your mind and prepare for sleep.
- Best consumed fresh, but can be stored in the fridge for up to 24 hours. Reheat before drinking.

Nature's Aspirin

Nature's Aspirin is an herbal remedy made from ingredients known for their anti-inflammatory and pain-relieving properties, offering a natural alternative to pharmaceutical painkillers.

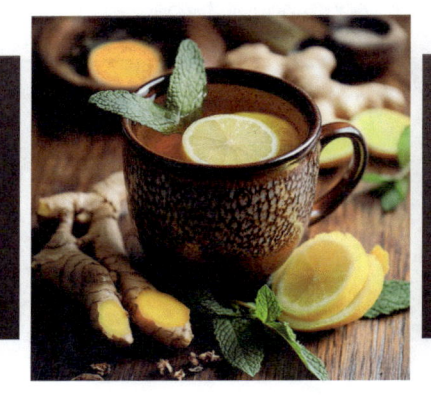

Ingredients:

- Willow Bark (1 teaspoon): Contains salicin, a compound similar to the active ingredient in aspirin, known for its ability to reduce pain and inflammation.
- Turmeric (1/2 teaspoon): A powerful anti-inflammatory, turmeric contains curcumin, which may help relieve pain associated with inflammation.
- Ginger (1/2 teaspoon): Known for its natural pain-relieving and anti-inflammatory effects, ginger can be used to ease discomfort.
- Peppermint (1/4 teaspoon): Contains menthol, which can help relax muscles and relieve tension, often used to ease headaches and migraines.
- Lemon Juice (1 tablespoon): Adds a refreshing taste and helps with digestion, further supporting the body's natural detoxification processes.

Instructions:

1. Boil 1 cup of water in a saucepan.
2. Add all the herbs and let them steep for 10-15 minutes.
3. Strain and pour into a mug. Add honey for sweetness if desired.

- Drink 1-2 times a day to help reduce inflammation and alleviate pain. Best taken for occasional aches and pains or as part of a holistic health routine.
- Best consumed fresh, but can be stored in the fridge for up to 24 hours.

Deep Sleep Banana Tea

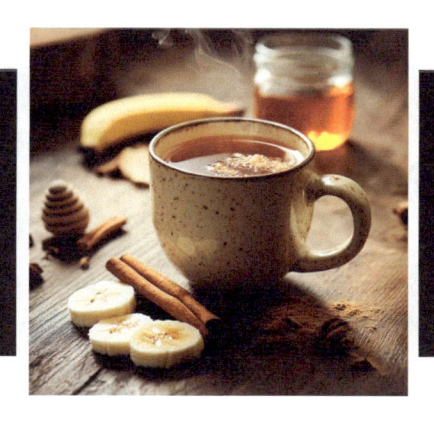

Deep Sleep Banana Tea is a soothing herbal remedy known for its calming effects, promoting relaxation and a restful night's sleep. This tea combines the natural sleep-supportive benefits of banana peel, magnesium, and other calming ingredients to ease the mind and body.

Ingredients:

- Banana Peel (1 peeled banana): The peel contains magnesium and potassium, which can help relax muscles and calm the nervous system.
- Cinnamon (1/4 teaspoon): Known for its calming properties, cinnamon also supports digestion and can enhance the soothing qualities of the tea.
- Nutmeg (1/4 teaspoon): A natural sedative, nutmeg promotes relaxation and helps induce sleep.
- Honey (optional, 1 teaspoon): Adds natural sweetness and may also help calm inflammation, supporting a restful sleep.

Instructions:

1. Boil 2 cups of water in a saucepan.
2. Slice the banana peel and add it to the water with cinnamon and nutmeg.
3. Let it simmer for 10-15 minutes to extract the beneficial properties from the peel.
4. Strain and pour into a mug. Add honey for sweetness if desired.
- Drink a cup of this tea about 30-60 minutes before bedtime to help ease into a peaceful sleep.
- Best consumed fresh, but can be stored in the fridge for up to 24 hours.

Soothing Herbal Soak

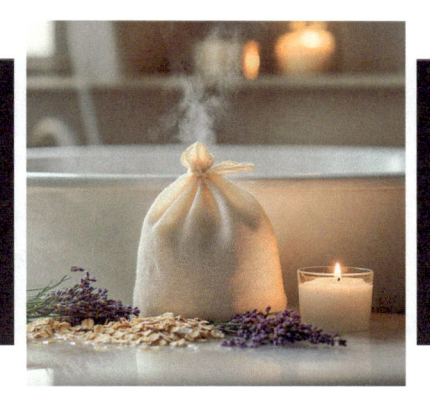

A soothing herbal soak is perfect for relieving stress, calming the mind, and relaxing sore muscles. This soak uses a blend of calming herbs to create a tranquil bath experience that nourishes both body and soul.

Ingredients:

- Lavender (1/2 cup): Known for its calming properties, lavender helps relieve stress, anxiety, and promotes relaxation.
- Chamomile (1/4 cup): A gentle, soothing herb that helps relax the body and mind, perfect for a peaceful soak.
- Epsom Salt (1 cup): Rich in magnesium, Epsom salt helps to relax muscles, reduce inflammation, and promote overall relaxation.
- Oatmeal (1/2 cup): Adds a skin-nourishing element, great for calming irritated skin.
- Rose Petals (1/4 cup, optional): Adds a touch of luxury and fragrance to the soak, enhancing the calming effect.

Instructions:

1. Combine all the dry ingredients in a small bowl.
2. Place the mixture in a muslin bag or cheesecloth, tying it securely.
3. Fill the bathtub with warm water and place the herbal bag under the running water to release the beneficial properties.
4. Soak for 20-30 minutes, allowing the herbs to relax your mind and body.
- Enjoy this soak as part of your evening self-care routine or after a long day for ultimate relaxation.
- Store the dry herbs in a cool, dry place in an airtight container until ready to use.

St. John's Wort and Linden Calming Infusion

This calming infusion combines the soothing properties of St. John's Wort and Linden flowers to promote relaxation, reduce stress, and support overall mental wellness. Ideal for unwinding after a busy day or before sleep.

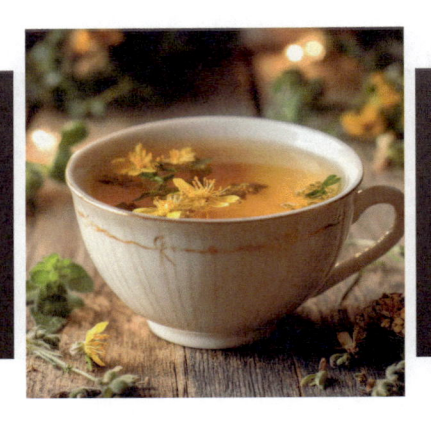

Ingredients:

- St. John's Wort (1 tablespoon): Known for its mood-lifting and anti-anxiety properties, it helps calm the nervous system and may support emotional balance.
- Linden Flowers (1 tablespoon): Gentle and relaxing, Linden is traditionally used to relieve stress, anxiety, and insomnia, while promoting relaxation.
- Honey (1 teaspoon): Adds natural sweetness and helps soothe the throat.
- Water (1 cup): To infuse the herbs.

Instructions:

1. Mix the St. John's Wort and Linden flowers in a cup of hot water.
2. Let the herbs steep for 10-15 minutes.
3. Strain the herbs and add honey, stirring until dissolved.

- Sip the infusion in the evening to promote relaxation and prepare for a restful sleep.
- Freshly prepare each time, as it's best consumed right after mixing.

Nature's Sedative

This calming blend is designed to gently soothe the nervous system, relieve tension, and promote a sense of peace and relaxation. With a combination of herbs known for their calming and sedative effects, it's the perfect remedy to unwind after a stressful day.

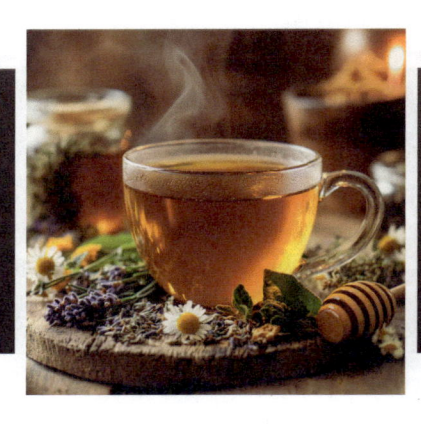

Ingredients:

- Valerian Root (1 tablespoon): Known for its powerful sedative properties, Valerian root is often used to promote deep relaxation and support better sleep.
- Chamomile Flowers (1 tablespoon): Chamomile is a well-known relaxant, helpful for reducing anxiety and easing into sleep.
- Lavender (1 teaspoon): Lavender's calming scent has been shown to reduce stress and anxiety while promoting relaxation.
- Honey (1 teaspoon): Adds natural sweetness and has soothing effects on the throat.
- Water (1 cup): Used to infuse the herbs.

Instructions:

1. Mix the valerian root, chamomile flowers, and lavender in a cup of hot water.
2. Let the herbs steep for 10-15 minutes.
3. Strain the herbs and add honey, stirring until dissolved.

- Drink slowly in the evening to calm the mind and prepare for a restful sleep.
- Freshly prepare each time, as it's best consumed right after mixing.

Stress-Free Elixir

This stress-relieving elixir combines calming herbs that are known to promote relaxation, balance mood, and reduce anxiety. It's perfect for unwinding after a long day or managing stress throughout the day.

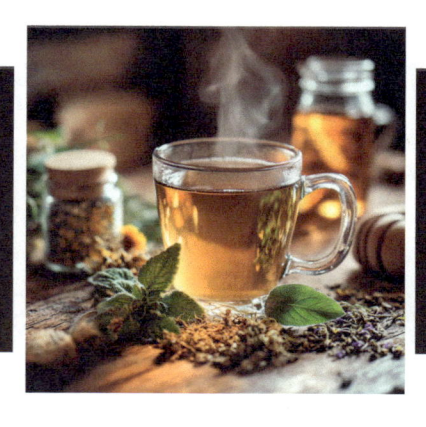

Ingredients:

- Ashwagandha Root (1 tablespoon): A powerful adaptogen that helps the body manage stress and anxiety while promoting a sense of calm.
- Lemon Balm (1 tablespoon): Known for its calming effects on the nervous system and its ability to reduce stress and improve mood.
- Passionflower (1 teaspoon): A soothing herb that promotes relaxation, reduces anxiety, and enhances sleep quality.
- Honey (1 teaspoon): A natural sweetener that adds a touch of comfort and helps to soothe the digestive system.
- Water (1 cup): Used to infuse the herbs and create a smooth elixir.

Instructions:

1. Mix the ashwagandha root, lemon balm, and passionflower in a cup of hot water.
2. Let steep for 10-15 minutes.
3. Strain the herbs and add honey, stirring until dissolved.

- Drink slowly in the morning or before bed to promote relaxation and stress relief.
- Freshly prepare each time, as it's best consumed right after mixing.

Stress Relief Herbal Candle

This calming herbal candle blend is designed to reduce stress and promote relaxation. Made with essential oils and herbs known for their soothing properties, this candle creates a peaceful atmosphere in your home.

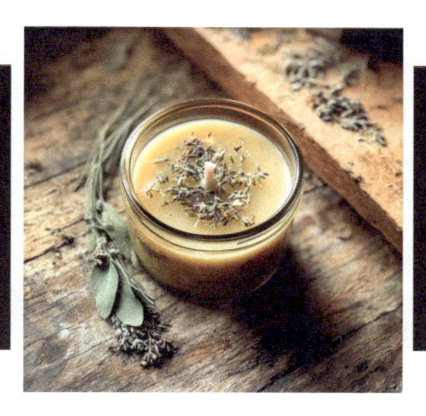

Ingredients:

- Lavender Essential Oil (10-15 drops): Known for its calming properties, lavender promotes relaxation and reduces stress.
- Chamomile Essential Oil (10 drops): Soothes nerves, alleviates anxiety, and encourages rest.
- Sage (dried leaves): Known for its purifying properties, sage clears negative energy and promotes mental clarity.
- Beeswax (1 cup): A natural base that helps the candle burn cleanly and releases a subtle, natural scent.
- Coconut Oil (2 tablespoons): Used to bind the wax and ensure a smooth, even burn.

Instructions:

1. Melt the beeswax and coconut oil in a double boiler.
2. Once melted, remove from heat and add the essential oils and dried sage.
3. Pour the mixture into a candle mold or jar, ensuring the wick is centered.
4. Allow the candle to cool and harden completely.

- Light the candle when you need to unwind or relax, such as during meditation, before bedtime, or during a bath.
- Keep in a cool, dry place when not in use.

At-Home Sedative to Alleviate Panic Attacks

This calming at-home remedy is designed to alleviate the symptoms of panic attacks and reduce anxiety. It uses a blend of natural herbs and ingredients known for their ability to soothe the nervous system, calm the mind, and promote relaxation.

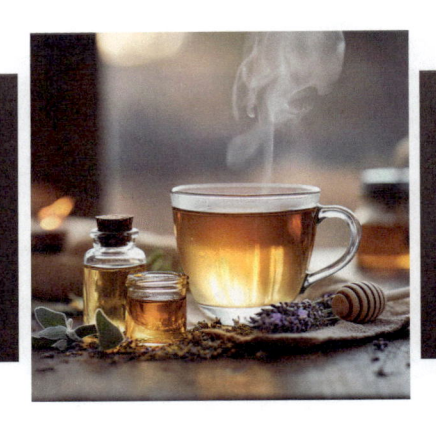

Ingredients:

- Lavender Essential Oil (10 drops): Lavender has been studied for its calming effects, making it ideal for reducing anxiety and stress.
- Chamomile Tea (1 cup): Chamomile has mild sedative effects and Is often used to calm nerves and promote relaxation.
- Lemon Balm (1 tablespoon, dried): Known for its ability to ease anxiety and promote a sense of calm.
- Valerian Root (1 teaspoon, dried): A powerful herb used for its sedative properties to ease stress and induce relaxation.
- Honey (1 teaspoon): Used to sweeten the tea and promote relaxation.

Instructions:

1. Brew chamomile tea and add lemon balm.
2. Add valerian root to the tea and let steep for 10-15 minutes.
3. Strain the herbs and stir in honey for added sweetness.
4. Drink the tea slowly, taking deep breaths as you sip.

- Sip slowly during a panic attack or as a preventative measure during stressful times.
- Freshly prepare each time for the most effective results.

Restorative Tablets to Ease Mental Pressure

This blend of natural ingredients is designed to ease mental pressure, reduce anxiety, and promote clarity. The soothing properties of these herbs help calm an overstressed mind, improve focus, and restore emotional balance.

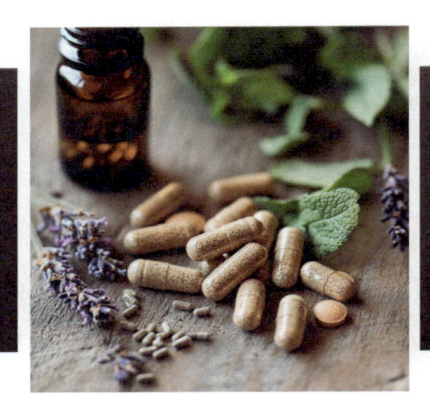

Ingredients:

- Ashwagandha (500 mg): Known for its adaptogenic properties, ashwagandha helps the body cope with stress and anxiety.
- Lemon Balm (200 mg): Provides a calming effect and has been traditionally used to reduce anxiety and improve mood.
- Rhodiola (200 mg): A powerful herb used to improve mental clarity, reduce fatigue, and enhance resilience to stress.
- Magnesium (100 mg): Helps reduce tension and supports proper brain function, alleviating mental fatigue.
- Lavender Essential Oil (5 drops): Known for its calming and relaxing effects, lavender helps promote mental relaxation and reduce stress.

Instructions:

1. In a small bowl, mix the powdered herbs (ashwagandha, lemon balm, rhodiola, and magnesium).
2. Add 5 drops of lavender essential oil to the mix, stirring gently.
3. Form into small tablets, pressing the mixture into molds or rolling by hand.
4. Allow tablets to dry completely before storing in a cool, dry place.

- Take 1 tablet daily, especially during times of stress, or as needed to relieve mental pressure.
- Store in an airtight container for up to 3 weeks.

"Sweet Dreams" Herbal Pillow

This soothing herbal pillow is designed to help you unwind and achieve a peaceful night's sleep. Filled with calming herbs, it releases a gentle aroma that promotes relaxation, reduces anxiety, and prepares your body for restful slumber.

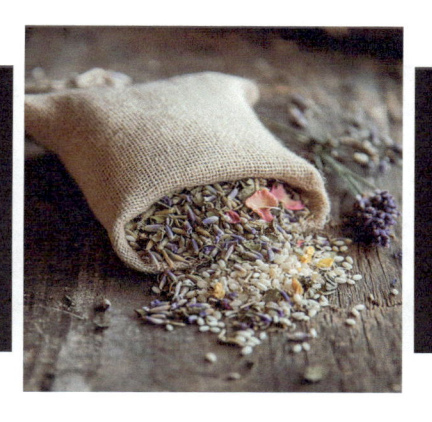

Ingredients:

- Lavender (2 tablespoons): Known for its calming and sleep-promoting properties, lavender helps ease tension and anxiety.
- Chamomile (1 tablespoon): A gentle herb that helps relax the nervous system and induces sleep.
- Lemon Balm (1 tablespoon): Reduces stress and promotes a sense of calm.
- Hops (1 tablespoon): Helps with insomnia and acts as a natural sedative.
- Rose Petals (1 tablespoon): Adds a delicate fragrance that soothes and calms the mind.
- Rice or Buckwheat Hulls (for filling): A soft base to hold the herbs in place and create a comfortable pillow.

Instructions:

1. Mix the dried herbs (lavender, chamomile, lemon balm, hops, and rose petals) in a bowl.
2. Add the rice or buckwheat hulls as the filling for the pillow.
3. Sew a small cloth pouch or pillowcase and fill it with the herbal mixture, making sure it's securely closed.
4. Place the pillow under your pillowcase or near your bed to enjoy the calming scent throughout the night.
- Place the herbal pillow on your bed or near your head while sleeping.
- Store in a cool, dry place, and refresh the herbs by adding a few drops of lavender essential oil every few weeks to maintain the aroma.

Herbal Sleeping Pills

These natural herbal sleeping pills are designed to help promote deep, restful sleep without the use of harsh chemicals. Crafted with a blend of calming herbs, these pills can assist in alleviating stress, easing tension, and preparing your body for a peaceful night's sleep.

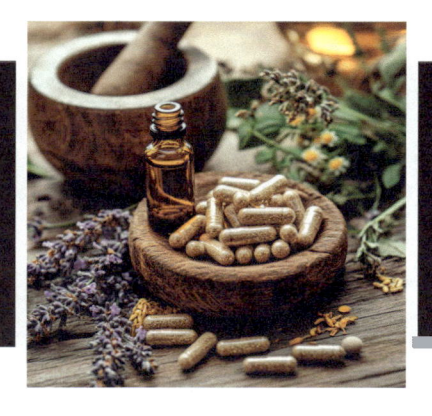

Ingredients:

- Valerian Root (1 teaspoon): Known for its sedative effects, valerian root is one of the most effective herbs for promoting sleep and reducing anxiety.
- Chamomile (1 teaspoon): Helps to relax the nervous system and induce sleep, commonly used for its calming effects.
- Lemon Balm (1 teaspoon): Reduces stress and anxiety, calming the mind and body for restful sleep.
- Passionflower (1 teaspoon): Used to treat insomnia, passionflower helps calm the mind and promote relaxation.
- Lavender Essential Oil (few drops): Known for its soothing properties, lavender oil helps calm nerves and promote a restful night's sleep.

Instructions:

1. In a small bowl, mix together the dried valerian root, chamomile, lemon balm, and passionflower.
2. Grind the herbs into a fine powder using a mortar and pestle or a spice grinder.
3. Add a few drops of lavender oil to the powdered herbs, stirring until well combined.
4. Fill small capsules (size 0 or 00) with the herbal mixture.
- Store the herbal sleeping pills in an airtight container, and consume within 3 months
- Take 1-2 capsules approximately 30 minutes before bedtime to promote relaxation and support restful sleep.

Bath Salt Mix for Relaxation

This soothing bath salt mix is a perfect way to unwind and de-stress after a long day. The combination of Epsom salt, essential oils, and natural botanicals helps to relax the muscles, calm the mind, and promote deep relaxation.

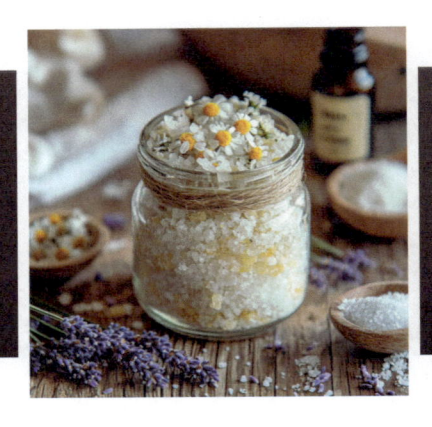

Ingredients:

- Epsom Salt (1 cup): Known for its muscle-relaxing properties, Epsom salt is rich in magnesium, which can ease tension and promote relaxation.
- Sea Salt (1/2 cup): Helps detoxify the skin and enhance the relaxing effects of the Epsom salt.
- Lavender Essential Oil (10-15 drops): Known for its calming and stress-reducing effects, lavender oil helps to promote deep relaxation.
- Chamomile Flowers (2 tablespoons, dried): A natural relaxant, chamomile helps calm the mind and soothe the nervous system.
- Baking Soda (1 tablespoon): Softens the water and can help relieve any skin irritation or discomfort during the bath.

Instructions:

1. In a large bowl, mix the Epsom salt, sea salt, and baking soda together.
2. Add the dried chamomile flowers and stir to combine.
3. Drop in the lavender essential oil and stir again to ensure even distribution.
4. Store the bath salt mix in a glass jar with a tight-fitting lid.
- Add 1/2 to 1 cup of the bath salt mix to warm bath water. Stir the water to dissolve the salts and allow them to infuse the bath with their soothing properties.
- Keep in a cool, dry place, and use within 6 months for the best results.

Kava Extract to Unwind & Get Relief

Kava is a traditional herb known for its calming effects on the mind and body. It is often used to promote relaxation, reduce anxiety, and ease stress, making it ideal for a soothing at-home remedy.

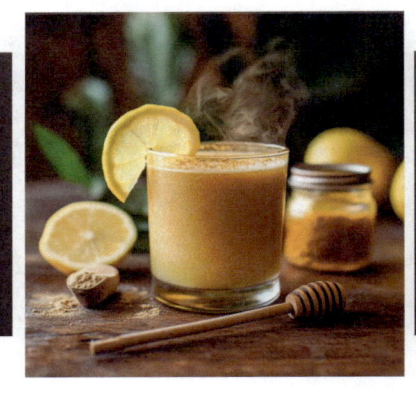

Ingredients:

- Kava Extract (1 teaspoon): The active compound kavalactones in kava have sedative and anxiolytic effects, helping to calm the mind and ease stress.
- Honey (1 teaspoon): Adds sweetness and can help soothe the throat, while also providing mild anti-inflammatory properties.
- Lemon Juice (1 tablespoon): Provides a refreshing citrus burst and adds vitamin C to support overall well-being.
- Water (1 cup): Acts as a base to dilute the kava extract and balance the flavors.

Instructions:

1. Mix the kava extract and honey in a cup of warm water.
2. Stir well to dissolve the honey.
3. Add the lemon juice and stir again.

- Sip the mixture slowly in the evening to promote relaxation and ease tension.
- Prepare fresh each time, as it's best enjoyed right after mixing.

The Legal Narcotic You Can Make at Home

Kava or Valerian root is often used to reduce anxiety and promote relaxation it's considered "legal narcotics" due to their calming properties that can help with anxiety, stress, and sleep disorders. These herbs can be safely used at home in various forms, like extracts, teas, or tinctures, but they are non-addictive and legally available.

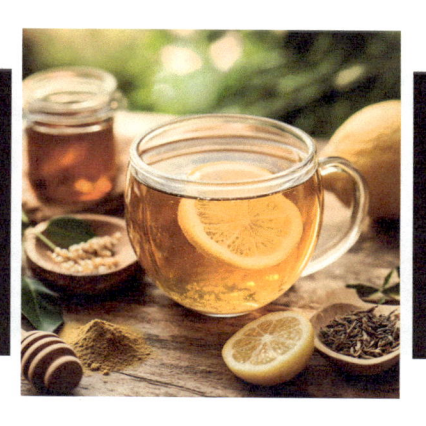

Ingredients:

- Kava Extract (1 teaspoon): Known for its ability to calm nerves and reduce anxiety, kava extract can help you unwind and alleviate stress.
- Valerian Root (1 teaspoon, dried): Valerian is often used as a natural sedative for its mild calming effects that aid sleep and reduce restlessness.
- Lemon Juice (1 tablespoon): Enhances the flavor and supports detoxification.
- Honey (1 teaspoon): Adds natural sweetness and soothing qualities.

Instructions:

- Mix kava extract and valerian root in a cup of warm water.
- Stir in honey until dissolved and add lemon juice.
- Stir well.

- Sip slowly in the evening or before bed to promote relaxation and aid sleep.
- Best freshly prepared, as the active ingredients are most potent when consumed soon after mixing.

Happiness Hormones Booster

This uplifting blend is designed to naturally support the production of the body's happiness hormones—serotonin, dopamine, and endorphins. These hormones help improve mood, alleviate stress, and foster a sense of well-being. Using natural herbs and ingredients that boost your body's ability to generate these vital chemicals can help you feel more energized and happy.

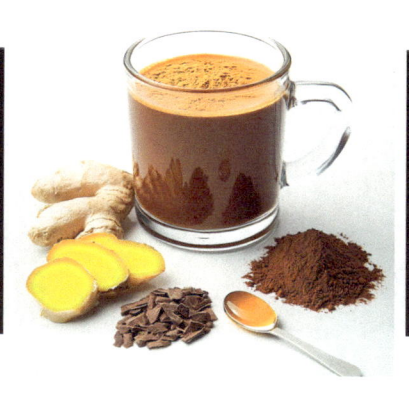

Ingredients:

- Cacao Powder (1 tablespoon): cacao helps stimulate the production of endorphins, which improve mood and reduce stress.
- Turmeric (1/2 teaspoon): Contains curcumin, which is known to promote the release of serotonin and dopamine, helping to improve overall mood and mental clarity.
- Ginger (1 teaspoon, fresh or powdered): Ginger is known for its ability to reduce inflammation and boost dopamine levels, contributing to improved mental health.
- Honey (1 teaspoon): A natural sweetener that provides a quick source of energy and helps boost serotonin levels.
- Coconut Oil (1 tablespoon): Supports healthy brain function and balances hormone levels, aiding in mood regulation.

Instructions:

1. Mix all ingredients in a glass of warm water.
2. Stir well until honey dissolves.

- Sip slowly in the morning or when you need an energy and mood boost.
- Freshly prepare each time, as it's best consumed right after mixing.

Worry Relieving Tincture

This soothing tincture is crafted with herbs known to support relaxation and relieve worry, helping to calm the nervous system.

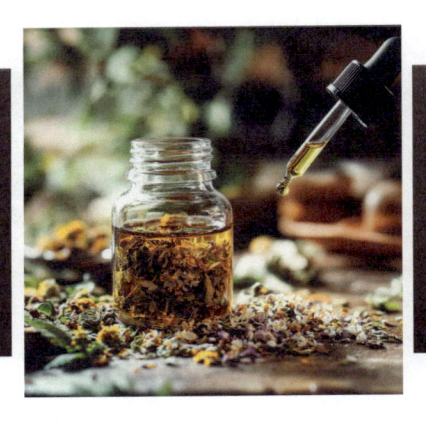

Ingredients:

- Lemon Balm (1 tablespoon, dried): Known for its calming effects, often used to relieve anxiety and promote sleep.
- Chamomile (1 tablespoon, dried): Traditionally used for its soothing properties to help ease nervous tension.
- Passionflower (1/2 tablespoon, dried): Helps to calm the mind and reduce feelings of worry.
- Apple Cider Vinegar (1/2 cup): Acts as the base to extract herbal compounds.

Instructions:

1. Place all herbs in a glass jar and pour in the apple cider vinegar.
2. Seal the jar tightly and store in a cool, dark place for 2-4 weeks, shaking daily.
3. Strain out the herbs and transfer the liquid to a dropper bottle.

- Take 15-20 drops in water up to twice daily for calming support.
- Store in a cool, dark place. The tincture should last for up to a year.

Lemon Balm and Skullcap Relaxing Tisane

This calming tisane blend combines lemon balm and skullcap, two herbs known for their soothing properties. It is ideal for reducing anxiety, promoting restful sleep, and easing stress after a long day.

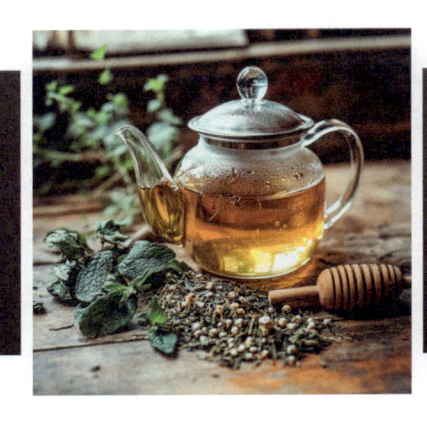

Ingredients:

- Lemon Balm (1 tablespoon dried): Known for its mild sedative properties, lemon balm helps relieve stress, anxiety, and digestive discomfort.
- Skullcap (1 tablespoon dried): A calming herb that promotes relaxation, reduces nervous tension, and helps improve sleep quality.
- Hot Water (1 cup): To brew the herbs and release their healing properties.
- Honey (optional, 1 teaspoon): For a natural sweetener and added soothing properties.

Instructions:

1. Place lemon balm and skullcap in a teapot or mug.
2. Pour hot water over the herbs and steep for 5-10 minutes.
3. Strain the herbs and add honey if desired. Stir well.

- Sip slowly in the evening to unwind and relax before bed or during moments of stress. Freshly prepare each time for maximum potency. Drink immediately after brewing.

Peaceful Mind Drops

These calming drops use gentle, herbal ingredients to support relaxation, relieve stress, and bring a sense of peace to the mind.

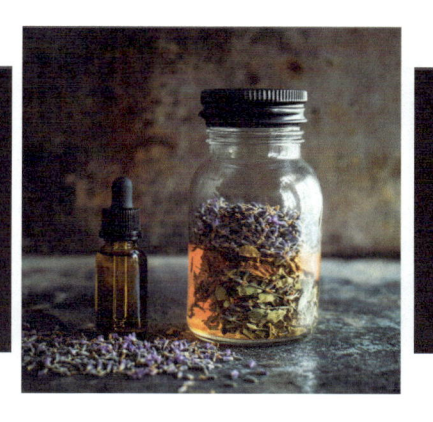

Ingredients:

- Lavender (1 tablespoon, dried): Known for its soothing aroma, lavender helps calm the nervous system and reduce stress.
- Valerian Root (1/2 tablespoon, dried): Commonly used to promote relaxation and improve sleep quality.
- Lemon Balm (1 tablespoon, dried): Helps relieve anxiety and bring emotional balance.
- Apple Cider Vinegar (1/2 cup): Acts as the base to extract and preserve the herbal properties.

Instructions:

1. Place the dried herbs in a glass jar
2. Add the apple cider vinegar.
3. Seal the jar and store in a cool, dark place for 2-4 weeks, shaking daily.
4. Strain the herbs and transfer the liquid into a dropper bottle.
5. Store the liquid in a dropper bottle for easy use.

- Take 10-15 drops up to three times a day, or as needed, to promote mental clarity, ease anxiety, and restore peace of mind. Keep in a cool, dark place. It can be stored for up to 6 months.

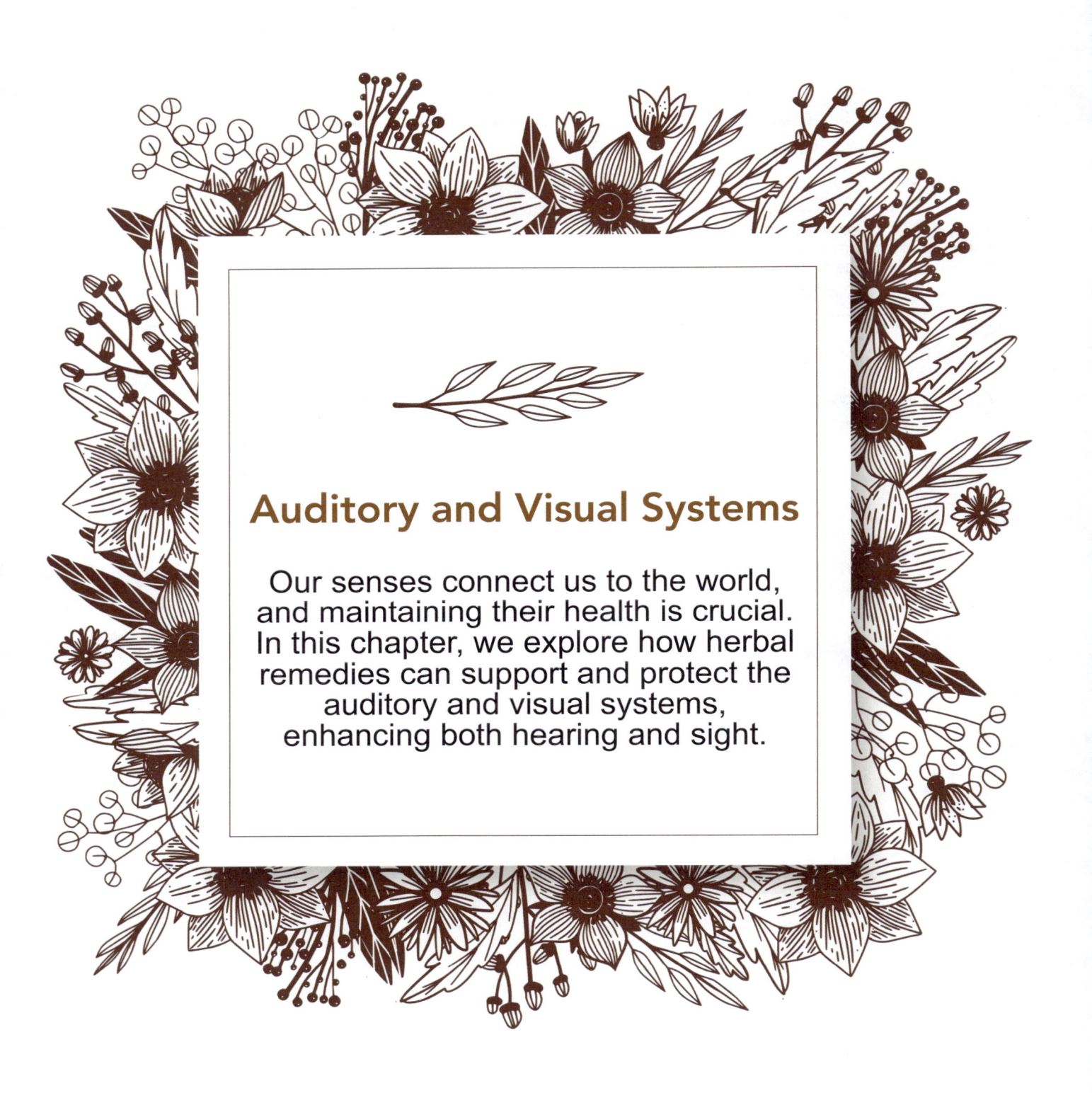

Auditory and Visual Systems

Our senses connect us to the world,
and maintaining their health is crucial.
In this chapter, we explore how herbal
remedies can support and protect the
auditory and visual systems,
enhancing both hearing and sight.

Tinnitus Relief Glycerite

This soothing glycerite is designed to help reduce the symptoms of tinnitus and ear ringing. It is made from herbs known to support nerve health, reduce inflammation, and calm the auditory system, offering a natural remedy to manage the discomfort of persistent ear ringing.

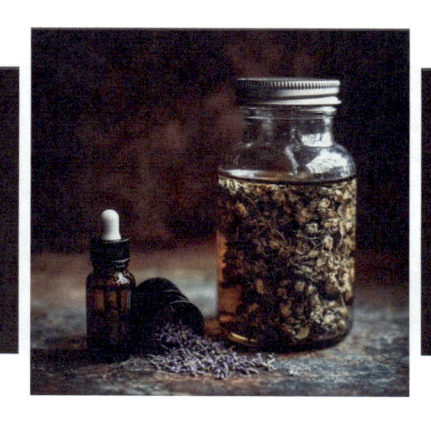

Ingredients:

- Hops (1 tablespoon, dried): Known for its calming effects on the nervous system, hops can help relieve the stress and anxiety that may accompany tinnitus.
- Lavender (1 tablespoon, dried): Lavender has anti-inflammatory properties and can help calm nerve irritability, potentially reducing tinnitus symptoms.
- Glycerin (1/4 cup): Glycerin acts as a preservative and helps to extract the beneficial compounds from the herbs.
- Distilled Water (1/4 cup): Used to dilute the glycerin, creating a balanced solution.

Instructions:

1. Combine hops and lavender in a glass jar.
2. Pour in glycerin and distilled water, mixing the ingredients well.
3. Seal the jar and let it steep in a cool, dark place for 2-3 weeks, shaking it occasionally.
4. After the steeping period, strain the liquid through a fine mesh or cheesecloth to remove the plant matter.
- Take 1-2 dropperfuls of the glycerite up to 3 times a day, either directly under the tongue or diluted in water or tea. Store in a cool, dark place. Use within 6 months for the best potency.

Vertigo Relief Herbal Infusion

This soothing herbal oil blend is crafted to help ease the symptoms of vertigo and dizziness. With a combination of herbs that support circulation and reduce inflammation, this oil can be massaged into the scalp or neck to provide relief from the discomfort of vertigo.

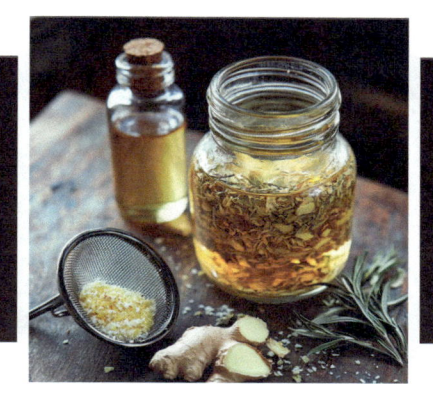

Ingredients:

- Ginger (1 tablespoon, dried or fresh): Ginger has been shown to help with nausea and dizziness, which are often associated with vertigo. It also has anti-inflammatory properties.
- Peppermint (1 tablespoon, dried or fresh): Peppermint oil is known for its ability to stimulate circulation and provide a cooling sensation that can help relieve dizziness.
- Rosemary (1 tablespoon, dried or fresh): Rosemary has circulatory benefits and is often used to treat vertigo and dizziness by improving blood flow to the head and neck.
- Carrier Oil (such as coconut or olive oil, 1/4 cup): A base oil to dilute the essential oils and make them safe for topical application.

Instructions:

1. Combine ginger, peppermint, and rosemary in a glass jar.
2. Add the carrier oil and stir well to mix the herbs.
3. Seal the jar and let the herbs infuse in the oil for 1-2 weeks in a cool, dark place, shaking occasionally.
4. After the steeping period, strain out the herbs using a fine mesh or cheesecloth.
- Gently massage a few drops of the oil onto the back of the neck, temples, or scalp as needed to alleviate vertigo symptoms. Keep in a cool, dark place for up to 6 months.

Parsley Tinnitus Relief Patch

This natural remedy uses parsley, known for its anti-inflammatory and circulation-boosting properties, to create a soothing patch for tinnitus. It may help reduce the ringing in the ears caused by poor circulation or inflammation.

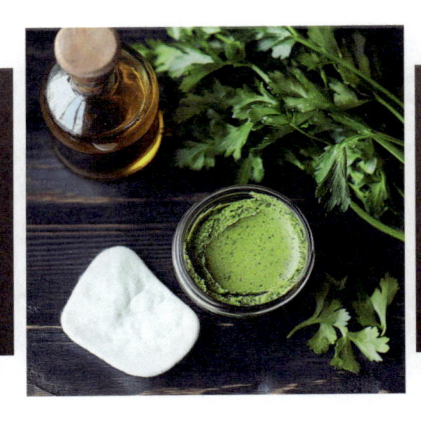

Ingredients:

- Parsley (fresh or dried): Known for its detoxifying and anti-inflammatory properties, parsley can help with circulation and inflammation, which may alleviate symptoms of tinnitus.
- Olive Oil (1 tablespoon): Acts as a base to help the parsley adhere to the skin and provides additional anti-inflammatory benefits.
- Gauze or cotton pads: To apply the parsley mixture to the skin.

Instructions:

1. Crush fresh parsley or use dried parsley and mix it with olive oil to create a paste.
2. Apply the paste to a cotton pad or gauze.
3. Place the patch gently over the affected ear area for about 20 minutes.
4. Remove and rinse the area with warm water.

- Apply 1-2 times a day for relief from tinnitus symptoms.
- Store unused parsley paste in an airtight container in the refrigerator for up to 3 days.

Herbal Ear Relief Compress

This soothing ear compress combines the anti-inflammatory properties of herbs like chamomile and ginger to help reduce ear pain and inflammation. Ideal for soothing irritation from ear infections or sinus congestion, this compress helps promote circulation and provides natural relief.

Ingredients:

- Chamomile Tea (1 bag or 1 tablespoon dried): Chamomile is known for its anti-inflammatory and soothing properties, ideal for easing ear discomfort.
- Ginger Root (1 teaspoon fresh, grated or powdered): Ginger helps with circulation and has anti-inflammatory properties that may assist in reducing swelling and pain.
- Warm Water (1 cup): Acts as the base for the compress and aids in applying the remedy to the ear.
- Cloth or Cotton Pad: To apply the compress directly to the ear.

Instructions:

1. Brew chamomile tea with the dried flowers or tea bag and steep for 5-10 minutes.
2. Add grated ginger or ginger powder to the tea and stir well.
3. Soak a cloth or cotton pad in the warm infusion, making sure it is not too hot.
4. Apply the soaked cloth or cotton pad to the affected ear for 10-15 minutes, re-soaking if necessary to maintain warmth.

- Apply the compress 1-2 times a day for ear discomfort due to inflammation or infection.
- Store any leftover herbal tea in the refrigerator for up to 2 days, but always use fresh for compresses.

Natural Antibacterial Eye Drops

These homemade antibiotic eye drops are crafted from natural ingredients that are known for their ability to fight bacteria and soothe irritated eyes. Ideal for mild infections, this remedy may help reduce symptoms of conjunctivitis, eye irritation, or minor eye infections.

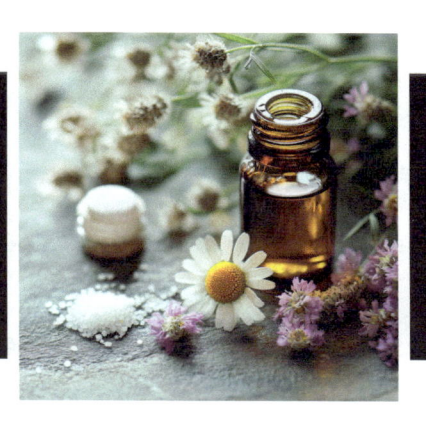

Ingredients:

- Chamomile Tea (1 tablespoon dried flowers or 1 tea bag): Chamomile is known for its anti-inflammatory and antibacterial properties, which can help to calm irritated eyes.
- Echinacea (1 teaspoon dried or extract): Echinacea is believed to have antimicrobial properties, useful for fighting infection.
- Salt (1/4 teaspoon): Salt helps in drawing out bacteria and soothing inflammation.
- Water (1 cup): Acts as the base to create a solution for eye drops.

Instructions:

1. Boil 1 cup of water and steep chamomile flowers or tea bag for 10 minutes to create a tea infusion.
2. Add 1 teaspoon of Echinacea and stir well. Let the mixture cool to room temperature.
3. Once cool, strain the tea into a clean bottle or eye dropper container, and add salt to the mixture. Stir until the salt dissolves completely.
4. Store in a sterilized container, and refrigerate.
- Place 1-2 drops in each affected eye, up to 3 times a day for relief from irritation or infection.
- Keep the eye drops in the refrigerator and use within 3-5 days for optimal effectiveness. Always discard if there are signs of contamination.

Soothing Calendula and Rose Eye Rinse

This soothing and anti-inflammatory eye wash combines calendula and rose water to relieve irritation, reduce redness, and promote eye health. Calendula has well-known anti-inflammatory and antimicrobial properties, while rose water calms and refreshes the eyes, offering relief from discomfort.

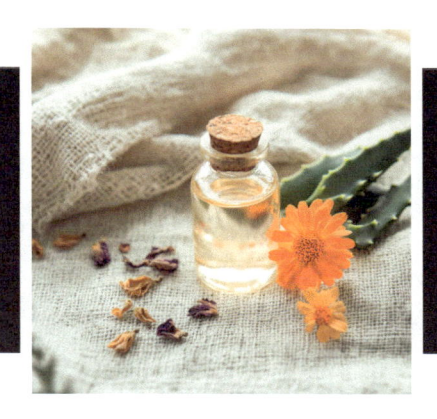

Ingredients:

- Calendula Flowers (1 tablespoon dried): Known for its healing properties, calendula helps soothe irritated eyes, reduce swelling, and prevent infection.
- Rose Water (2 tablespoons): Helps reduce redness and provides calming relief for tired or inflamed eyes.
- Distilled Water (1/2 cup): Acts as a neutral base to dilute the herbal infusion and ensure it's safe for the eyes.
- Optional: Aloe Vera Gel (1 teaspoon): Adds extra soothing qualities, especially for dry or sensitive eyes.

Instructions:

1. Boil the distilled water and steep the calendula flowers in it for 10-15 minutes to create a potent herbal infusion.
2. Strain the flowers and let the infusion cool completely to room temperature.
3. Stir in the rose water and aloe vera (if using).
4. Transfer the mixture into a clean container with a tight lid.
- Use an eye dropper or small clean cup to gently rinse the eyes with the cooled infusion. Blink a few times to help distribute the liquid across the eye.
- Keep the eye wash in the refrigerator and use within 3-4 days. Discard any unused solution if there are signs of contamination.

Cooling Cucumber and Aloe Eye Mask

This cooling and soothing mixture of aloe vera and cucumber is designed to reduce puffiness, refresh tired eyes, and hydrate the delicate skin around the eyes. Both aloe vera and cucumber have natural anti-inflammatory properties, making this blend perfect for calming and rejuvenating fatigued eyes.

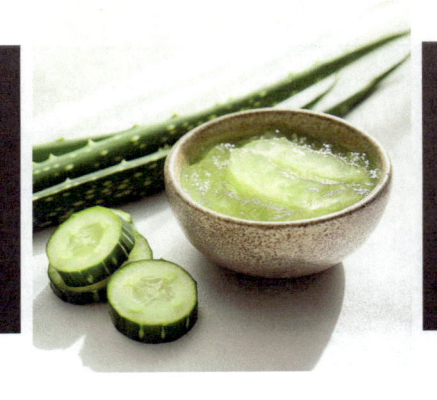

Ingredients:

- Aloe Vera Gel (1 tablespoon): Known for its hydration and soothing properties, aloe vera can reduce puffiness and irritation around the eyes.
- Cucumber (1/4 cucumber, peeled and chopped): Contains antioxidants and silica, which help reduce swelling and refresh tired skin.
- Rose Water (1 teaspoon, optional): Adds additional soothing and cooling properties, beneficial for relieving redness and irritation.

Instructions:

1. Blend the peeled cucumber until smooth, then strain to extract the juice.
2. Mix the cucumber juice with aloe vera gel in a small bowl.
3. Optionally, add rose water for extra calming benefits.
4. Apply a small amount of the mixture to a cotton pad or directly to the skin around the eyes, avoiding direct contact with the eyes.
- Leave it on for 10-15 minutes, then gently rinse with cool water.
- Apply this mixture as a cooling eye mask whenever your eyes feel tired, puffy, or irritated.

Bilberry Vision Support Tonic

Bilberries, rich in anthocyanins, are known for their ability to support eye health and improve circulation to the eyes, making this glycerite an excellent natural remedy for enhancing night vision and overall eye function.

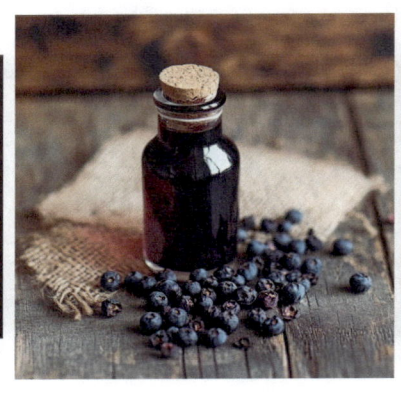

Ingredients:

- Bilberry (1 tablespoon, dried or fresh): Contains powerful antioxidants that support eye health, improve blood circulation, and enhance night vision.
- Vegetable Glycerin (1/4 cup): A natural solvent used to extract the beneficial compounds from the bilberry while preserving them in a sweet, easy-to-take form.
- Filtered Water (1/4 cup): Used to dilute the glycerin and aid in the extraction process.

Instructions:

1. In a clean jar, combine the bilberries and vegetable glycerin.
2. Add filtered water to the jar and stir the mixture well.
3. Seal the jar and let it sit in a cool, dark place for 2 weeks, shaking it daily.
4. After 2 weeks, strain out the berries using a fine mesh strainer or cheesecloth.
5. Transfer the strained glycerite into a clean bottle or jar for storage.
- Take 1-2 teaspoons of the bilberry glycerite daily, either in water or as is, to support eye health and improve circulation.
- Store in an airtight container in a cool, dark place for up to 6 months.

Ginkgo Biloba Vision & Circulation Boost Tincture

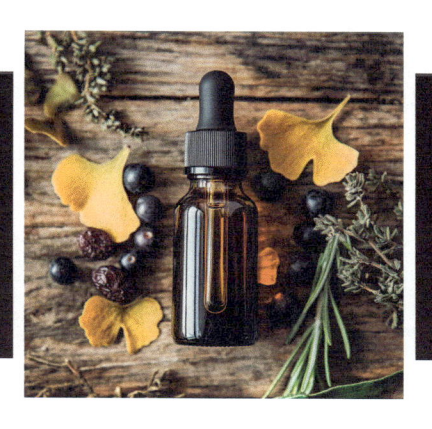

Ginkgo Biloba is a well-known herb that helps enhance blood circulation, including to the eyes, supporting retinal health and improving visual function. This tincture is formulated to support eye health, improve circulation to the eyes and ears, and promote overall visual and auditory wellness.

Ingredients:

- Ginkgo Biloba (1 tablespoon, dried): Known for increasing blood flow and supporting eye and ear health.
- Bilberry (1 tablespoon, dried): Rich in antioxidants, helpful for night vision and reducing eye strain.
- Rosemary (1/2 tablespoon, dried): Improves circulation and acts as an antioxidant.
- Apple Cider Vinegar (1/2 cup): A non-alcoholic base to preserve the tincture and extract beneficial compounds.

Instructions:

1. Place the dried herbs in a glass jar and cover with apple cider vinegar.
2. Seal the jar, and store in a cool, dark place for 2-4 weeks, shaking daily.
3. Strain out the herbs and pour the liquid into a dropper bottle.
4. Store the tincture in a clean, airtight bottle.

- Take 10-15 drops in water once daily to support eye and auditory health.
- Keep the tincture in a cool, dark place for up to 6 months.

Eye-Guard Antioxidant Blend

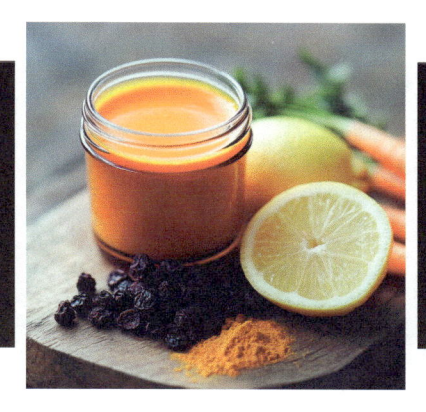

This antioxidant-rich infusion is designed to protect and nourish your eyes, using ingredients that are known for their protective effects against oxidative stress and for supporting overall eye health.

Ingredients:

- Bilberry (1 tablespoon, dried): Rich in anthocyanins, which have been shown to support eye health and protect against oxidative damage.
- Lutein (1 teaspoon, powdered): A powerful antioxidant that helps protect the eyes from harmful blue light and oxidative stress, promoting long-term eye health.
- Carrot Juice (1/4 cup): Packed with beta-carotene, which is converted into vitamin A to support healthy vision.
- Lemon Juice (juice of 1/2 lemon): Vitamin C from lemon aids in collagen production and strengthens the eye's lens and capillaries.

Instructions:

1. Combine the bilberry and lutein in a small jar or glass.
2. Add the carrot juice and lemon juice, mixing well.
3. Stir the mixture until all ingredients are thoroughly blended.
4. Drink immediately to enjoy the full benefits.

- Drink 1/2 cup daily to help protect your eyes from oxidative damage and improve circulation to the retina.
- Freshly prepare each time, as it's best consumed right after mixing for maximum nutrient retention.

Ear Relief Soothing Oil

This soothing ear oil blend helps to relieve discomfort caused by ear irritation, inflammation, and infections. It uses natural ingredients known for their antibacterial, anti-inflammatory, and soothing properties, offering a safe alternative to over-the-counter ear drops.

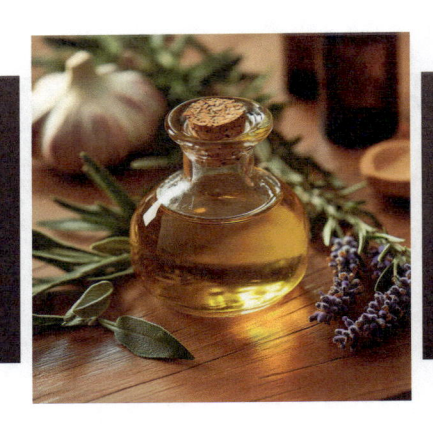

Ingredients:

- Garlic Oil (1 tablespoon): Garlic has natural antibacterial and antifungal properties that can help fight infections and reduce inflammation.
- Tea Tree Oil (2-3 drops): Known for its antimicrobial properties, tea tree oil can help treat ear infections and soothe irritation.
- Lavender Oil (2 drops): Lavender oil helps calm inflammation and reduce pain, while also promoting relaxation.
- Olive Oil (1/4 cup): Serves as a carrier oil to dilute essential oils, and it also soothes and moisturizes the ear canal.

Instructions:

1. Mix all ingredients in a small glass container.
2. Gently warm the mixture by placing the container in a bowl of warm water for a few minutes.
3. Using a clean dropper, apply a few drops of the oil mixture into the affected ear while lying on your side.
4. Let it sit for 5-10 minutes before draining excess oil.
- Apply 2-3 drops of the oil mixture to the affected ear once or twice a day until symptoms subside. Store in a cool, dark place. Use within 2-3 weeks for optimal freshness.

Ear Comfort Relief Spray

This custom ear spray is formulated to ease discomfort caused by ear aches and infections, combining natural ingredients known for their antimicrobial, anti-inflammatory, and soothing properties. It helps relieve pain, promote healing, and provide comfort during ear-related issues.

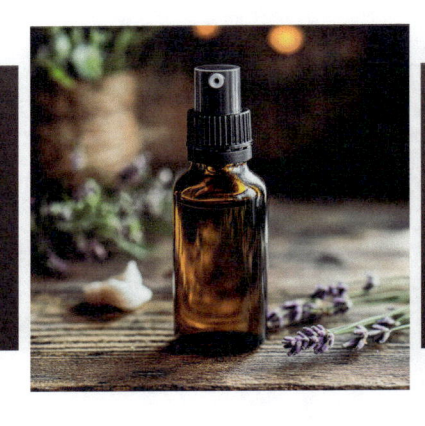

Ingredients:

- Garlic Oil (1 tablespoon): Known for its natural antibacterial and antifungal properties, garlic oil can help treat ear infections and reduce inflammation.
- Tea Tree Oil (5-6 drops): A powerful antimicrobial agent, tea tree oil helps combat infections and soothes irritated skin in the ear canal.
- Lavender Oil (3 drops): Lavender oil helps to reduce pain, calm inflammation, and promote relaxation.
- Witch Hazel (1/4 cup): Witch hazel has natural astringent properties that help cleanse and reduce swelling in the ear area.
- Distilled Water (1/4 cup): Used to dilute and mix the oils, ensuring the spray is gentle on the ear.

Instructions:

1. In a small spray bottle, combine garlic oil, tea tree oil, lavender oil, witch hazel, and distilled water.
2. Shake well before each use to ensure the ingredients are properly mixed.
3. Spray 1-2 spritzes directly into the ear canal, or spray onto a cotton ball and gently swab the inside of the ear.
- Use 1-2 spritzes up to twice a day to help relieve ear pain and discomfort. Store the spray in a cool, dark place. Use within 2 weeks for freshness.

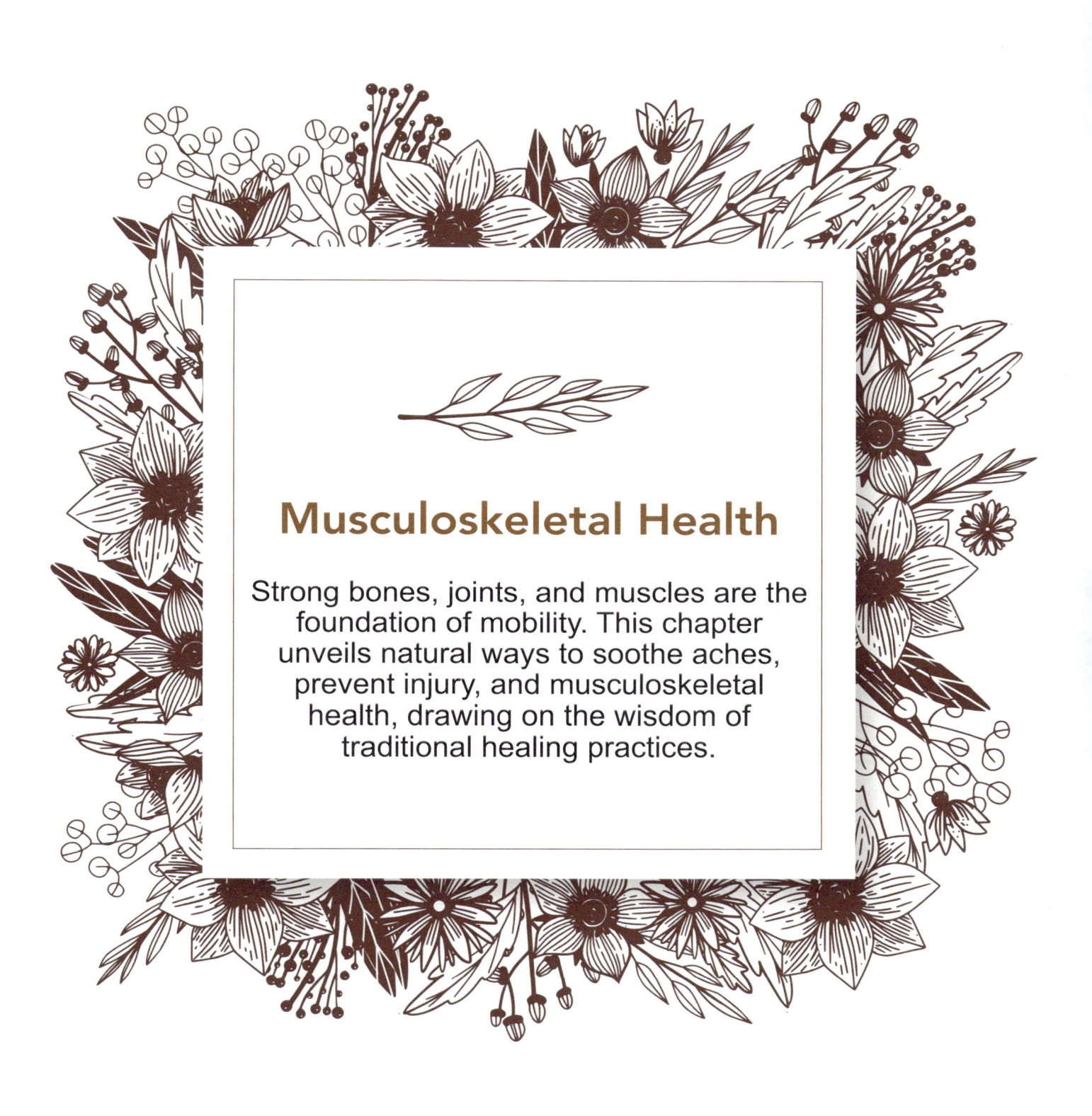

Musculoskeletal Health

Strong bones, joints, and muscles are the foundation of mobility. This chapter unveils natural ways to soothe aches, prevent injury, and musculoskeletal health, drawing on the wisdom of traditional healing practices.

Soothing Muscle & Joint Relief Balm

This natural pain relief balm combines the soothing and anti-inflammatory properties of essential oils and herbs to help alleviate muscle pain, headaches, or joint discomfort. It offers a homemade remedy with ingredients that are easily accessible and effective for targeted relief.

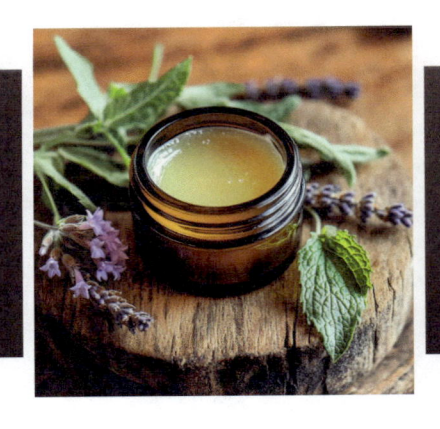

Ingredients:

- Arnica Oil (1 tablespoon): Known for its ability to reduce inflammation and pain, particularly in muscles and joints.
- Peppermint Oil (5-10 drops): Provides a cooling sensation and works to relieve tension and pain.
- Lavender Oil (5 drops): Helps with relaxation and also has pain-relieving properties.
- Coconut Oil (2 tablespoons): A carrier oil that helps dilute essential oils and moisturize the skin.
- Beeswax (1 tablespoon): Adds texture and helps the balm solidify, making it easy to apply.

Instructions:

1. Gently heat the coconut oil and beeswax in a double boiler until melted.
2. Once melted, remove from heat and stir in the arnica oil, peppermint oil, and lavender oil.
3. Pour the mixture into a small jar and let it cool completely to solidify.
- Apply a small amount of the balm to sore muscles, joints, or areas of discomfort. Massage gently to allow it to absorb.
- Store in a cool, dry place. The balm will last for up to 6 months when properly stored.

Herbal Pain Relief Infusion

This homemade pain-relief remedy uses traditional ingredients found in Amish medicine to help ease muscle pain, headaches, and inflammation. It combines the healing properties of herbs and essential oils known for their natural pain-relieving effects.

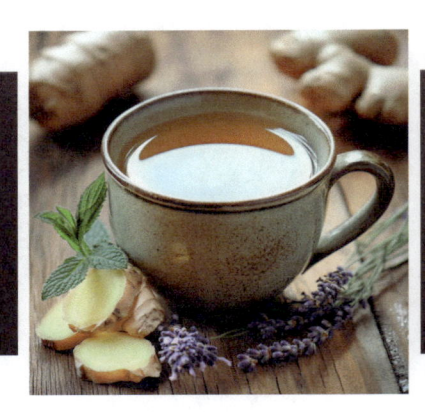

Ingredients:

- Willow Bark (1 tablespoon): Known as nature's aspirin, willow bark contains salicin, a compound similar to aspirin, making it effective for pain and inflammation.
- Ginger (1 teaspoon, dried or fresh): Offers anti-inflammatory properties and can help with muscle aches and pains.
- Peppermint Oil (5-10 drops): Provides a cooling sensation and helps relieve headaches and muscular pain.
- Lavender Oil (5 drops): lavender can help ease tension and reduce pain.
- Honey (1 teaspoon): Used to sweeten the remedy and has natural anti-inflammatory properties.

Instructions:

1. Boil 1 cup of water and steep the willow bark and ginger in the hot water for 10 minutes.
2. Strain the herbs, then add the peppermint and lavender essential oils and honey to the infusion.
3. Stir well and allow the infusion to cool to room temperature.
- Drink 1 cup of the infusion daily, preferably in the morning or when experiencing pain. The combination of willow bark and ginger provides a gentle yet effective way to manage discomfort.
- Store the infusion in an airtight container in the refrigerator for up to 2-3 days. Reheat gently before use if needed.

Joint & Cartilage Soothing Balm

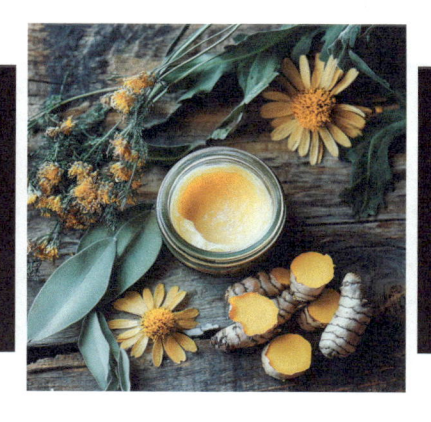

This soothing cream is designed to promote joint and cartilage health. By combining natural anti-inflammatory herbs and oils, this cream can help with discomfort caused by conditions like osteoarthritis and muscle stiffness, supporting the repair and regeneration of cartilage over time.

Ingredients:

- Arnica Oil (1 tablespoon): Known for its anti-inflammatory properties, arnica oil helps reduce pain and swelling in joints and muscles.
- Turmeric Powder (1 teaspoon): Contains curcumin, which has powerful anti-inflammatory properties that can aid cartilage health.
- Coconut Oil (2 tablespoons): Serves as a base oil that also helps moisturize and soothe the skin while carrying the active ingredients deeper into the tissue.
- Eucalyptus Oil (5-7 drops): Offers a cooling sensation, which can help reduce joint stiffness and inflammation.
- Beeswax (1 tablespoon): Acts as a natural emulsifier, binding the ingredients together and providing a protective layer over the skin.

Instructions:

1. In a double boiler, gently melt the beeswax and coconut oil together.
2. Once melted, remove from heat and stir in the turmeric powder and arnica oil.
3. Add the eucalyptus oil, mixing well.
4. Pour the cream into a small jar or container and let it cool to room temperature.
- Apply a small amount of the cream to sore joints or areas of inflammation. Massage gently in circular motions for better absorption.
- Store in a cool, dry place. The cream can last up to 3 months if kept away from direct sunlight.

Comfrey & Lavender Muscle Relief Oil

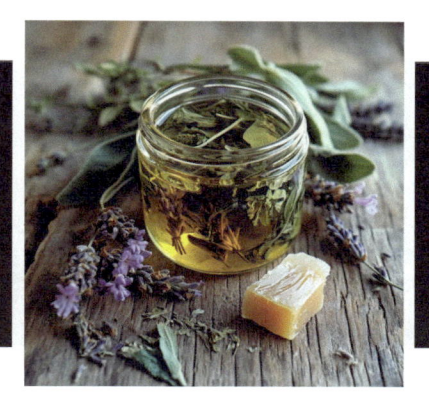

This soothing herbal oil blend combines the healing properties of comfrey and lavender, which are well-known for their ability to support joint health, ease muscle tension, and reduce inflammation. Comfrey's natural allantoin helps in tissue repair, while lavender provides a calming effect and reduces pain.

Ingredients:

- Comfrey Root or Leaf (1 tablespoon dried): Known for its tissue-healing properties and ability to soothe inflammation in joints and muscles.
- Lavender Oil (10 drops): Offers anti-inflammatory benefits and promotes relaxation.
- Olive Oil (1/4 cup): Serves as the base oil, helping to carry the active ingredients into the skin.
- Beeswax (1 teaspoon): Helps to thicken the oil and provides a protective barrier on the skin.

Instructions:

1. Gently heat olive oil in a double boiler, and add the comfrey root or leaf to infuse it for 1-2 hours.
2. Strain out the herb using a fine mesh sieve or cheesecloth, and return the infused oil to the boiler.
3. Stir in beeswax until fully melted and mixed.
4. Remove from heat, then add lavender essential oil.
5. Pour into a sterilized jar or bottle and allow to cool.
- Massage into sore or stiff joints and muscles to relieve pain and support healing.
- Store in a cool, dry place. This herbal oil can last up to 6 months if kept away from direct sunlight.

Collagen Boosting Herbal Elixir

This elixir combines nutrient-rich ingredients that support skin elasticity, hair growth, and overall joint health, providing an alternative to traditional collagen supplements. Packed with natural sources of vitamins and minerals, this blend boosts collagen production and provides the body with the tools needed for optimal skin and tissue repair.

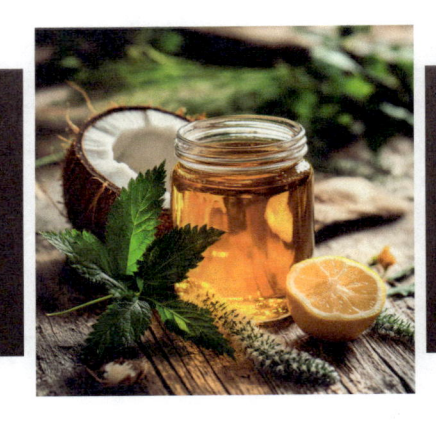

Ingredients:

- Horsetail Herb (1 tablespoon dried): Known for its silica content, which supports skin, hair, and nails by boosting collagen production.
- Nettle Leaf (1 tablespoon dried): Rich in minerals and vitamins, nettle helps to strengthen connective tissues and improve skin health.
- Vitamin C (1 teaspoon powdered or fresh juice of 1 lemon): Essential for collagen synthesis and skin repair.
- Ginger Root (1/2 teaspoon dried or fresh): Aids circulation and supports the body's ability to produce collagen.
- Coconut Oil (1 tablespoon): Provides healthy fats that promote skin hydration and elasticity.

Instructions:

1. Steep the horsetail herb and nettle leaf in hot water for 10-15 minutes.
2. Strain the herbs and add the ginger, Vitamin C (or lemon juice), and coconut oil to the infusion.
3. Stir well until the coconut oil is dissolved.
- Drink 1 cup daily to support skin health, hair growth, and joint flexibility.
- Store in the refrigerator for up to 3 days, and prepare fresh each time for optimal benefits.

Sports Relief Herbal Liniment

This herbal liniment can be a powerful aid in relieving pain and swelling associated with sports injuries and strains. It combines anti-inflammatory herbs and essential oils known for their muscle-soothing properties.

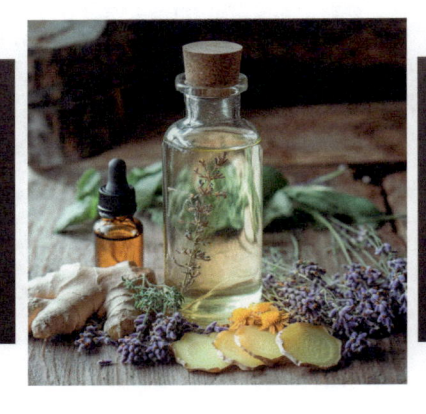

Ingredients:

- Arnica (1 tablespoon dried): A powerful herb often used for bruising, swelling, and muscle soreness. It helps reduce inflammation and promotes healing.
- Ginger (1 tablespoon fresh or dried): Known for its warming effects and ability to improve circulation, which helps to ease muscle tension and reduce pain.
- Lavender Essential Oil (10 drops): Calming and soothing for the skin, lavender essential oil is known to relieve muscle tension and promote relaxation.
- Eucalyptus Essential Oil (10 drops): A cooling oil that reduces inflammation, eases pain, and promotes circulation.
- Witch Hazel (1/2 cup): Used as a base, witch hazel provides a cooling and anti-inflammatory effect, helping to reduce swelling and pain.

Instructions:

1. Combine arnica and ginger in a glass jar.
2. Pour in witch hazel and add the essential oils.
3. Shake well and allow the mixture to infuse for 2-3 days in a dark place.
- Apply the liniment to the affected area 2-3 times a day, massaging it gently into the skin.
- Keep in a cool, dark place for up to 3 months. Shake before each use.

Grandma's Back Pain Relief Salve

This natural salve is designed to provide relief for sore, tense muscles and back pain. It combines warming, soothing, and anti-inflammatory ingredients like cayenne pepper, arnica, and eucalyptus to ease discomfort and promote circulation.

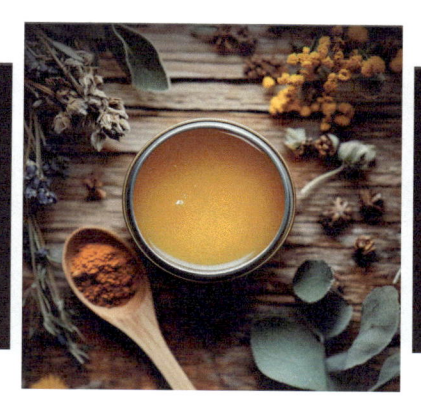

Ingredients:

- Cayenne Pepper (1 tablespoon): Known for its ability to ease pain and inflammation by stimulating blood flow.
- Arnica (1 tablespoon dried): Reduces swelling and bruising, commonly used for muscle pain and strains.
- Eucalyptus Essential Oil (10 drops): Known for its cooling and anti-inflammatory properties that help alleviate pain.
- Beeswax (2 tablespoons): Creates the salve's base, offering a protective barrier for the skin.
- Olive Oil (1/2 cup): Helps blend and infuse the active ingredients while nourishing the skin.

Instructions:

1. Melt beeswax and olive oil together in a double boiler.
2. Once melted, add arnica and cayenne, stirring until combined.
3. Remove from heat and allow it to cool slightly before adding eucalyptus oil. Stir to mix well.
4. Pour the mixture into jars or tins and allow it to cool completely before use.
- Massage a small amount onto affected areas of the back. Reapply as needed.
- Keep in a cool, dry place for up to 6 months.

Arthritis Relief Mobility Tincture

This soothing tincture blend is formulated to help maintain joint mobility and reduce discomfort related to arthritis. The combination of anti-inflammatory herbs works to support flexibility and relieve joint pain.

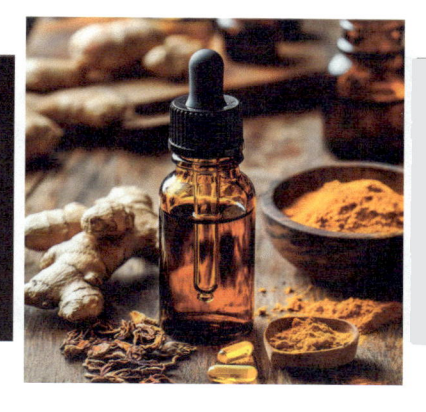

Ingredients:

- Turmeric (1 tablespoon, dried): Known for its strong anti-inflammatory properties, beneficial for easing joint stiffness and pain.
- Ginger Root (1 tablespoon, dried): Reduces inflammation and helps alleviate pain associated with arthritis.
- Devil's Claw (1 tablespoon, dried): Traditionally used for relieving arthritis and joint pain.
- Apple Cider Vinegar (1/2 cup): Acts as a preservative and enhances herb extraction without alcohol.

Instructions:

1. Combine the dried herbs in a glass jar and cover with apple cider vinegar.
2. Seal the jar and store in a cool, dark place for 2-4 weeks, shaking it daily.
3. Strain the mixture and transfer the liquid to a dropper bottle.
- Take 1-2 dropperfuls, 1-3 times a day, in a small amount of water or juice.
- Keep in a cool, dark place for up to 1 year.

Natural Joint Pain Relief Remedy

This remedy is designed to help reduce inflammation and alleviate joint pain using natural herbs with anti-inflammatory and pain-relieving properties.

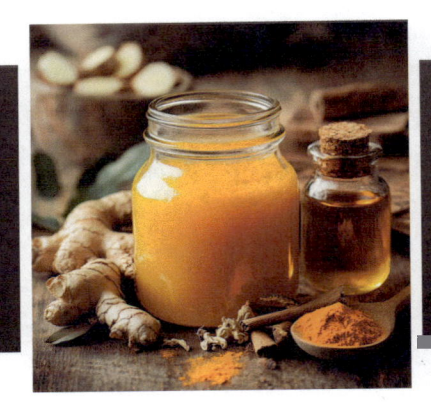

Ingredients:

- Turmeric (1 tablespoon, dried): Known for its strong anti-inflammatory properties, turmeric helps to reduce joint pain and swelling.
- Ginger (1 tablespoon, dried): Contains compounds that fight inflammation and improve circulation.
- White Willow Bark (1 tablespoon, dried): Often used for its pain-relieving effects, especially for joint and muscle pain.
- Cayenne Pepper (1/2 teaspoon): Contains capsaicin, which helps reduce pain and inflammation in joints.
- Apple Cider Vinegar (1 tablespoon): Known for its alkalizing properties, it helps balance the body and reduce inflammation.
- Honey (1 teaspoon): Used for its soothing properties and to balance the tartness of the vinegar.

Instructions:

1. Combine the turmeric, ginger, and white willow bark in a glass jar.
2. Add the cayenne pepper and apple cider vinegar.
3. Pour in hot water, stir well, and let the mixture steep for 10 minutes.
4. Strain the herbs out and stir in honey until fully dissolved.
- Drink 1 cup of this mixture twice daily for relief from joint pain.
- Freshly prepare each time, as it's best consumed right after mixing.

Herbal Poultice for Arthritis Pain Relief

This soothing poultice combines three herbs with anti-inflammatory properties to help reduce pain and swelling associated with arthritis.

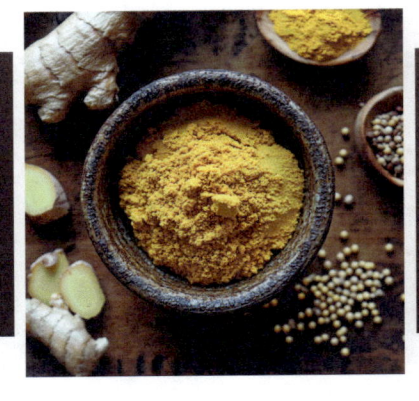

Ingredients:

- Turmeric (1 tablespoon, powdered): Known for its potent anti-inflammatory properties, turmeric helps reduce pain and inflammation in joints.
- Ginger (1 tablespoon, freshly grated): Contains compounds that can help alleviate joint pain and improve blood circulation.
- Mustard Seeds (1 tablespoon, ground): Mustard seeds have been used traditionally to ease pain and inflammation.

Instructions:

1. In a small bowl, mix the turmeric powder, grated ginger, and ground mustard seeds.
2. Add enough warm water to form a thick paste.
3. Apply the paste directly to the affected area, covering it with a cloth or bandage to keep the poultice in place.
4. Leave it on for about 20-30 minutes, then remove and rinse off with warm water.
- Apply the poultice to inflamed or painful joints twice daily for relief.
- Freshly prepare each time, as it's most effective when applied right away.

Herbal Anti-Inflammatory Tincture for Joint Relief

This potent anti-inflammatory tincture supports joint health by helping to reduce inflammation and relieve pain. A combination of herbs traditionally used for their anti-inflammatory and analgesic properties helps soothe joint discomfort and promote mobility.

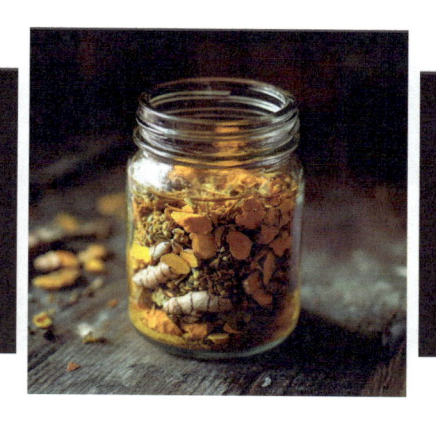

Ingredients:

- Turmeric Root (1 tablespoon, dried): Known for its powerful anti-inflammatory and pain-relieving properties, turmeric helps reduce joint inflammation.
- Ginger Root (1 tablespoon, dried): Acts as a natural pain reliever and anti-inflammatory, aiding in the reduction of swelling in the joints.
- Boswellia (1 teaspoon, dried): An herb known to help reduce inflammation and stiffness in the joints.
- Vegetable Glycerin (1 cup): A non-alcoholic base to extract and preserve the herbal properties.

Instructions:

1. Combine the dried turmeric root, ginger root, and boswellia in a glass jar.
2. Pour vegetable glycerin over the herbs, making sure they are fully covered.
3. Seal the jar tightly and let it steep in a cool, dark place for 2-3 weeks, shaking once a day.
4. After the steeping period, strain out the herbs using a fine mesh strainer or cheesecloth.
- Take 1-2 dropperfuls in water up to three times a day for joint pain relief and anti-inflammatory benefits.
- Store in a cool, dark place for up to one year. Always shake before use and make fresh batches as needed.

Soothing DIY Balm for Pain Relief and Skin Irritation

This DIY relieving balm is ideal for soothing sore muscles, alleviating joint pain, and calming skin irritations. With a combination of herbal ingredients, it's a natural and effective remedy.

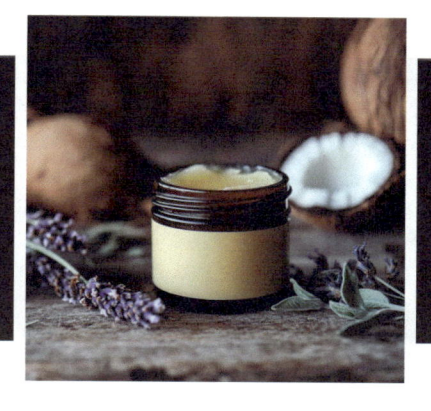

Ingredients:

- Beeswax (1/4 cup): Acts as a solidifying agent and offers a protective barrier for the skin.
- Coconut Oil (1/2 cup): Provides hydration and helps to carry the active ingredients into the skin.
- Arnica Oil (2 tablespoons): Known for its ability to reduce swelling and pain.
- Peppermint Essential Oil (10-15 drops): Offers a cooling effect and helps to reduce pain.
- Lavender Essential Oil (10-15 drops): Soothes the skin and calms inflammation.
- Eucalyptus Essential Oil (10-15 drops): Has anti-inflammatory and pain-relieving properties.

Instructions:

1. In a double boiler, melt the beeswax and coconut oil together until completely liquid.
2. Once melted, remove from heat and add the arnica oil.
3. Add the essential oils and mix well.
4. Pour the mixture into small tins or jars and allow it to cool and solidify.
- Apply a small amount to sore muscles, joints, or irritated skin. Massage gently to allow the balm to absorb.
- Keep in a cool, dry place for up to 6 months.

Pineapple & Turmeric Pain Relief Extract

This extract utilizes the natural pain-relieving and anti-inflammatory properties of pineapple, particularly its bromelain content. Bromelain has been shown to reduce inflammation and ease joint pain, making it an effective remedy for musculoskeletal discomfort.

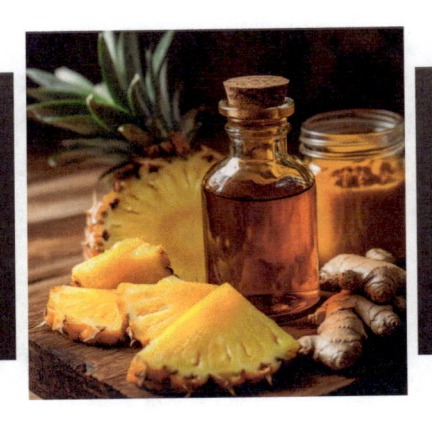

Ingredients:

- Fresh Pineapple (2 cups, chopped): Contains bromelain, which reduces inflammation and aids in the breakdown of proteins that cause swelling.
- Turmeric (1 tablespoon, dried): Known for its anti-inflammatory effects, helping to soothe joint pain and stiffness.
- Ginger (1 tablespoon, fresh or dried): Works as a natural pain reliever and reduces inflammation.
- Honey (1 tablespoon): Provides natural sweetness and soothing qualities, plus anti-inflammatory properties.
- Apple Cider Vinegar (1/2 cup): Enhances extraction and serves as a preservative.

Instructions:

1. Combine chopped pineapple, turmeric, and ginger in a glass jar.
2. Pour apple cider vinegar over the ingredients until covered.
3. Seal the jar and store in a cool, dark place for 2-3 weeks, shaking it daily.
4. Strain the mixture through a fine mesh strainer and transfer the liquid to a bottle.
- Take 1 teaspoon of the extract once or twice a day to help with muscle pain and inflammation. You can also apply the extract topically to affected areas for relief.

Backyard Serenity Capsules

These calming pills are a simple, natural remedy crafted with herbs from your backyard. This blend of calming botanicals can help alleviate stress, anxiety, and promote relaxation, making it a great choice for anyone looking for natural anxiety relief or sleep support.

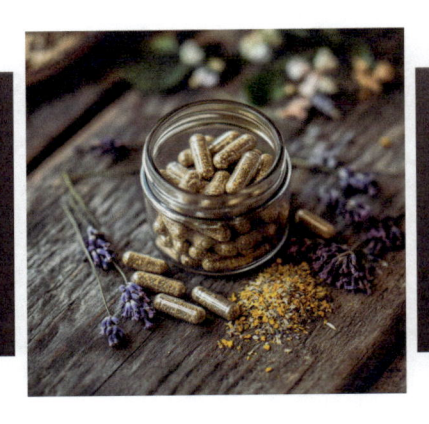

Ingredients:

- Chamomile (1 tablespoon, dried): Known for its relaxing and soothing properties, chamomile helps reduce stress and promotes sleep.
- Lavender (1 tablespoon, dried): A gentle herb that reduces anxiety and induces a sense of calm.
- Lemon Balm (1 tablespoon, dried): Helps to reduce nervousness and anxiety while calming the mind.
- Valerian Root (1/2 teaspoon, powdered): Known for its sedative effects, valerian root helps with sleep and muscle relaxation.

Instructions:

1. Combine all the herbs in a small mixing bowl.
2. Pour the mixture into a small jar and shake it gently.
3. Use a capsule machine to fill empty gelatin or vegetable capsules with the herbal mixture.
4. Once all the capsules are filled, seal them and store in an airtight container.
- Take 1-2 pills as needed for calming effects. They can be taken before bedtime or anytime anxiety arises.
- Keep in a cool, dry place for up to 6 months.

Magnesium Relief Cream for Leg Cramps

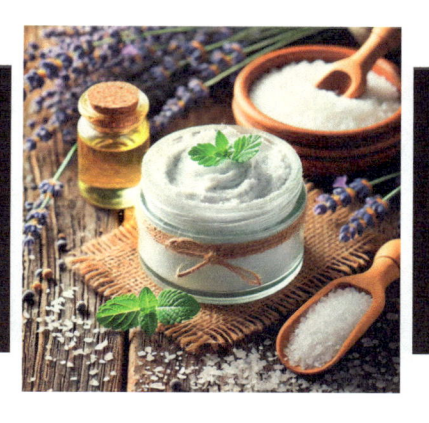

This soothing magnesium rub is a natural remedy to alleviate leg cramps and muscle tension. Magnesium is known for its muscle-relaxing properties, making it effective in easing cramps and promoting muscle relaxation.

Ingredients:

- Magnesium Chloride Flakes (1/2 cup): Known for its ability to relax muscles and ease cramps.
- Coconut Oil (1/4 cup): A soothing base for the rub, also moisturizes the skin.
- Lavender Essential Oil (10 drops): Adds a calming scent and promotes muscle relaxation.
- Peppermint Essential Oil (5 drops): Provides a cooling sensation to soothe discomfort.

Instructions:

1. In a small bowl, combine the magnesium chloride flakes with coconut oil.
2. Stir until well-mixed. The mixture may have a gritty texture due to the magnesium flakes.
3. Add the essential oils and stir again until evenly distributed.
4. Transfer the mixture into a glass jar or airtight container for storage.
- Gently massage the rub onto the legs, focusing on areas prone to cramping or tension. Use before bedtime for relaxation.
- Keep in a cool, dry place. The rub can be stored for up to 3 months.

Fermented Red Clover Elixir for Bone Health

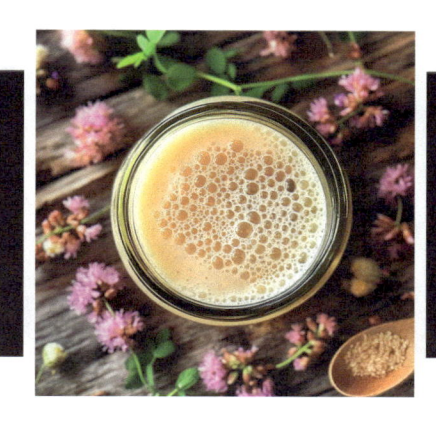

This fermented red clover preparation is designed to support bone health by harnessing the beneficial properties of the herb, which contains isoflavones that can help with bone density and overall skeletal strength. Fermentation not only enhances the absorption of these compounds but also provides a rich source of probiotics, which can aid in the absorption of minerals critical for bone health.

Ingredients:

- Red Clover (1 cup dried or fresh): Known for supporting bone health through its isoflavones, which mimic estrogen, promoting healthy bone metabolism.
- Water (2-3 cups): For fermenting the herbs.
- Probiotic Starter Culture (1 tablespoon): Can be from a previous batch of fermented foods, like kefir grains or a probiotic supplement.

Instructions:

1. Place the red clover into a clean glass jar.
2. Add enough water to cover the clover completely, leaving an inch of space at the top.
3. Stir in the probiotic starter culture until fully dissolved.
4. Cover with a cloth or lid and let ferment at room temperature for 3-7 days, stirring daily.
5. Once fermentation is complete, strain out the herb and transfer the liquid to a glass bottle for storage.
- Consume 1 tablespoon daily, mixed with water or tea, to support bone health.
- Keep refrigerated for up to 2 weeks.

Soothe & Heal Dandelion Salve

This homemade dandelion salve is a natural remedy that harnesses the healing power of dandelion, known for its anti-inflammatory and pain-relieving properties. It can be applied to sore muscles and joints for soothing relief.

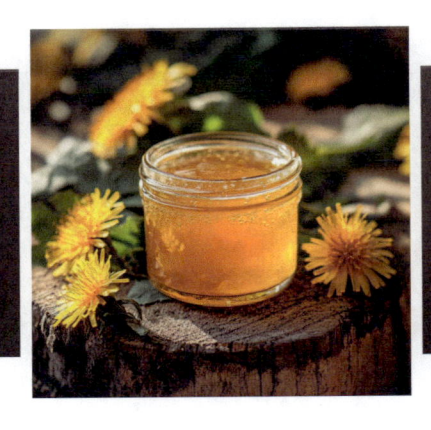

Ingredients:

- Dandelion flowers (1/4 cup, dried or fresh): Known for reducing inflammation, dandelion is used to alleviate muscle and joint pain.
- Olive or coconut oil (1/2 cup): Acts as a carrier oil to infuse the medicinal properties of dandelion into the skin.
- Beeswax (2 tablespoons): Helps solidify the salve and provides a protective barrier on the skin.
- Optional essential oils (10-15 drops): Lavender or peppermint for added soothing effects and a calming fragrance.

Instructions:

Infuse dandelion flowers in the oil by placing them in a jar and covering with olive or coconut oil. Heat gently in a double boiler for 1-2 hours, or leave in a sunny spot for 1-2 weeks.

Strain the flowers from the oil.

Melt beeswax in a double boiler and mix it with the infused oil.

Stir in essential oils (if using) and pour into jars. Let it cool to solidify.

- Massage into sore muscles and joints as needed for relief.
- Store in a cool, dry place. It will last for up to 6 months.

Nourishing Watercress Bone Broth for Joint Health

Watercress is a powerhouse herb packed with essential nutrients that support bone and joint health. This easy-to-make broth is designed to harness the healing properties of watercress, garlic, ginger, and bone broth to promote joint strength, reduce inflammation, and nourish your bones.

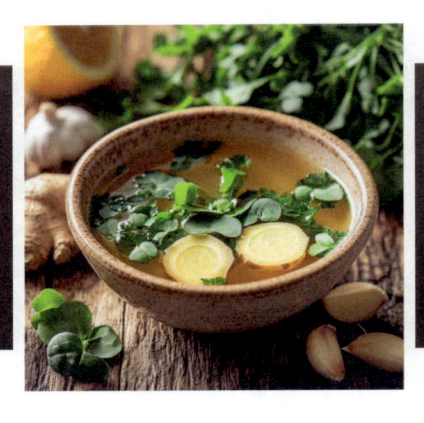

Ingredients:

- Watercress (1 cup, fresh): Rich in vitamin C, calcium, and iron, which are essential for bone density and joint health.
- Garlic (2 cloves, minced): helps with anti-inflammatory and circulation-boosting.
- Ginger (1-inch piece, sliced): A natural anti-inflammatory that helps reduce joint pain and stiffness.
- Bone Broth (2 cups): Contains collagen and essential minerals that strengthen joints and bones.
- Lemon Juice (1 tablespoon): Supports collagen production and adds a burst of vitamin C for overall joint health.

Instructions:

1. Bring the bone broth to a simmer in a pot.
2. Add garlic and ginger, letting them infuse the broth for 5-10 minutes.
3. Add watercress and simmer for another 5 minutes to allow the nutrients to infuse.
4. Stir in lemon juice and remove from heat.
5. Optionally, strain the broth to remove solids before serving.

- Drink this nourishing broth 2-3 times a week to promote joint health and strengthen bones.
- Refrigerate for up to 3 days or freeze for future use.

Green Boost Juice for Bone Health

This nutrient-packed juice is designed to support bone health, rich in vitamins and minerals that contribute to stronger bones and improved bone density. Combining green vegetables with calcium-rich fruits and herbs, it provides an easy and delicious way to nourish your body.

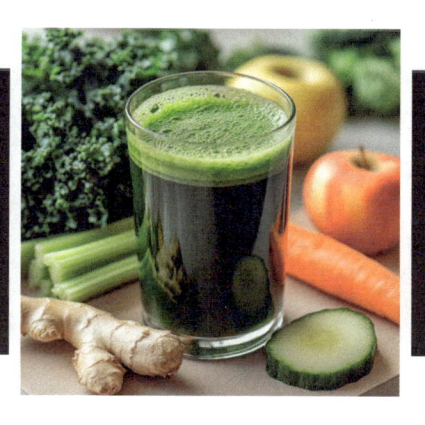

Ingredients:

- Kale (1 cup): Packed with calcium and vitamin K, crucial for bone health and strength.
- Carrot (1 large): Rich in vitamin A and beta-carotene, supporting overall bone density.
- Celery (2 stalks): Contains minerals like calcium and magnesium that help with bone and joint health.
- Apple (1, cored): Adds sweetness and vitamin C, promoting collagen production.
- Lemon Juice (1 tablespoon): Boosts vitamin C intake, aiding in collagen synthesis for bone flexibility.
- Ginger (1-inch piece, optional): Known for its anti-inflammatory properties, it can reduce joint pain associated with bone issues.

Instructions:

1. Juice all the ingredients (kale, carrot, celery, apple, ginger) together.
2. Add lemon juice and stir well.
3. Pour into a glass and enjoy immediately.
- Drink daily to support healthy bones and joints.
- Best consumed fresh, but can be stored in the refrigerator for up to 24 hours.

Cabbage Wraps for Joint Relief

Cabbage has long been used for its anti-inflammatory properties, particularly when applied topically. When used as a compress, cabbage leaves can help reduce swelling and ease pain in affected areas such as the knees, ankles, or elbows.

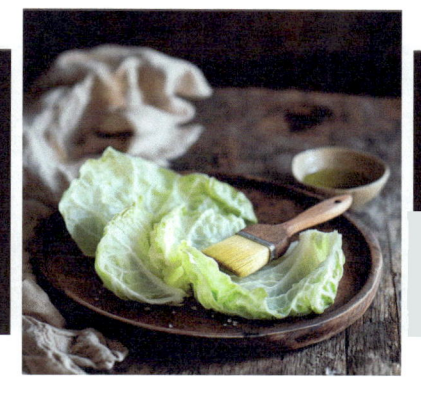

Ingredients:

- Cabbage (1 large head): Known for its anti-inflammatory properties, cabbage helps reduce swelling and soothes joints.
- Olive Oil (1 tablespoon, optional): To help enhance the cabbage's anti-inflammatory effect and add extra soothing qualities.

Instructions:

1. Remove several large cabbage leaves from the head.
2. Cut out the tough, central vein of the leaves to make them more pliable.
3. Gently heat the cabbage leaves in a warm oven for a few minutes or steam them.
4. If desired, rub olive oil lightly over the cabbage leaves for added soothing.
5. Place the warmed cabbage leaves on the affected area, wrapping them snugly like a "sock."
6. Leave them on for about 20-30 minutes, allowing the cabbage to cool as it draws out inflammation.
- Apply these cabbage "socks" to areas affected by joint pain or inflammation and leave them on for up to 30 minutes.
- Fresh cabbage leaves can be kept in the fridge, but prepare the compress each time for best results.

Pine Needle Infusion for Joint and Muscle Relief

Pine needles have been used in herbal medicine for centuries due to their potent anti-inflammatory and analgesic properties. Infusing pine needles into oil creates a soothing remedy that can help reduce pain and inflammation in joints, making it a great option for those dealing with conditions like arthritis or rheumatism.

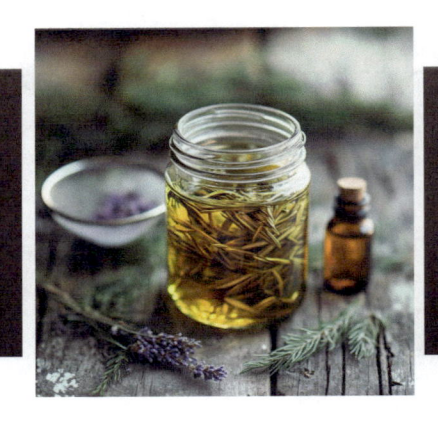

Ingredients:

- Pine Needles (1 cup, fresh or dried): Known for their anti-inflammatory and pain-relieving properties, pine needles help reduce joint pain and swelling.
- Olive Oil (2 cups): A great carrier oil that helps infuse the pine needle properties and acts as a moisturizer.
- Optional: Essential Oils (5-10 drops): You can add a few drops of essential oils such as lavender or eucalyptus for added soothing effects.

Instructions:

1. Place the fresh or dried pine needles into a clean glass jar.
2. Pour olive oil over the pine needles, ensuring they are fully submerged.
3. Seal the jar tightly and place it in a warm, sunny spot for 1-2 weeks, shaking it gently once a day to encourage the infusion.
4. After 1-2 weeks, strain the oil through a fine mesh strainer or cheesecloth to remove the pine needles.
5. If desired, add essential oils
- Apply the infused oil to affected areas, gently massaging it into sore joints and muscles.
- Store in a cool, dark place for up to 6 months.

Willow Bark Soothing Soak for Pain and Inflammation

Willow bark is known for its natural pain-relieving and anti-inflammatory properties due to the presence of salicin, a compound similar to aspirin. Incorporating it into bath salts allows for soothing relief from inflammation, muscle aches, and joint pain, making it an ideal remedy for those dealing with conditions like arthritis or chronic pain.

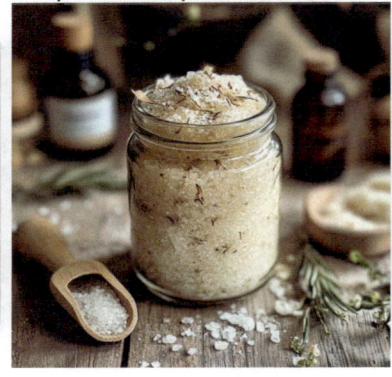

Ingredients:

- Willow Bark Powder (1/4 cup): Contains salicin, which helps reduce inflammation and provides natural pain relief.
- Epsom Salt (1 cup): Known for its muscle-relaxing properties and ability to reduce inflammation.
- Sea Salt (1/2 cup): Helps to detoxify the skin and soothe sore muscles.
- Baking Soda (1/4 cup): Soothes the skin and enhances the effects of the salts.
- Essential Oils (optional, 5-10 drops): You can add soothing oils like lavender, eucalyptus, or peppermint to enhance relaxation and add a pleasant fragrance.

Instructions:

1. In a bowl, combine willow bark powder, Epsom salt, sea salt, and baking soda.
2. Stir the ingredients until well mixed.
3. Add any essential oils of your choice and stir again.
4. Store the bath salts in an airtight container.
- Add 1-2 cups of the bath salts to your warm bath. Soak for at least 20-30 minutes to allow the salts and willow bark to soothe and reduce inflammation.
- Keep in a cool, dry place for up to 6 months.

Herbal Pain-Relief Patch with Willow Bark and Turmeric

These natural pain-relief patches combine the power of plants that mimic the effects of ibuprofen, offering a soothing alternative for muscle pain, joint discomfort, or inflammation. The patch works by allowing the body to absorb the beneficial properties of anti-inflammatory herbs directly through the skin.

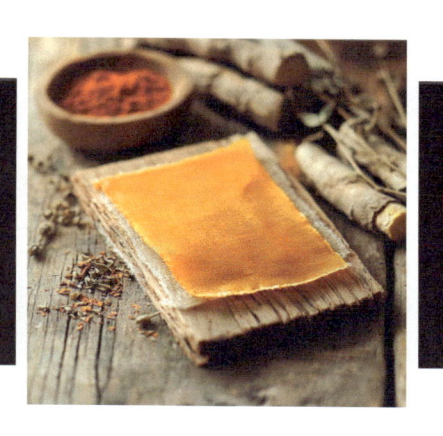

Ingredients:

- Willow Bark Powder (2 tbsps): Contains salicin, which has pain-relieving and anti-inflammatory properties, acting like natural ibuprofen.
- Turmeric Powder (1 tbsp): Known for its strong anti-inflammatory and antioxidant effects.
- Cayenne Pepper (1 tbsp): Contains capsaicin, which helps improve blood circulation and alleviates pain.
- Beeswax (1 tbsp): Acts as a base for the patch and helps it adhere to the skin.
- Coconut Oil (2 tbsps): A carrier oil that soothes the skin and allows better absorption of the active ingredients.
- Cloth or Gauze Strips: Used as the base material for the patch.

Instructions:

1. In a double boiler, melt the beeswax and coconut oil together.
2. Once melted, stir in the willow bark powder, turmeric, and cayenne pepper until well combined.
3. Pour the mixture over a cloth or gauze strip and let it harden into a patch.
4. Allow the patch to cool and solidify completely before use.
- Apply the patch to the area of discomfort. Leave it on for 1-2 hours, or as needed for relief.
- Store unused patches in a cool, dry place for up to 3 months.

Fibromyalgia Soothing Herbal Tea Blend

This herbal blend combines calming and anti-inflammatory herbs known for their ability to soothe fibromyalgia-related pain, reduce inflammation, and promote relaxation. The herbs work synergistically to alleviate discomfort, improve circulation, and provide overall relief for those experiencing chronic pain.

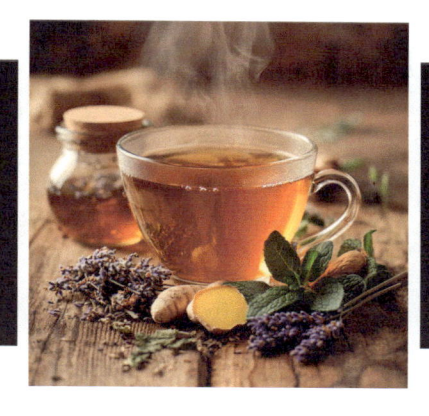

Ingredients:

- Turmeric Root (1 tbsp, dried or fresh): Contains curcumin which helps reduce pain and inflammation, common symptoms of fibromyalgia.
- Lavender (1 tbsp, dried): Known for its calming properties, lavender helps reduce stress and promote relaxation, which is essential for fibromyalgia sufferers.
- Ginger (1 tbsp, dried or fresh): Offers warming properties that help ease muscle pain and improve circulation.
- Peppermint (1 tbsp, dried): Provides a cooling sensation and works as a mild pain reliever.
- Chamomile (1 tbsp, dried): Known for its calming and anti-inflammatory effects, chamomile can help relax muscles and reduce pain.
- Honey (1 tbsp): Natural sweetener that also has anti-inflammatory and soothing properties.

Instructions:

1. Combine all the dried herbs in a bowl.
2. Boil water and pour it over the herbs, allowing them to steep for 5-10 minutes.
3. Strain the herbs out and stir in honey to sweeten the infusion.
- Sip slowly throughout the day, particularly when pain levels flare up. This soothing tea can be consumed hot or cold, depending on preference.
- Prepare fresh each time, as it's best consumed soon after brewing.

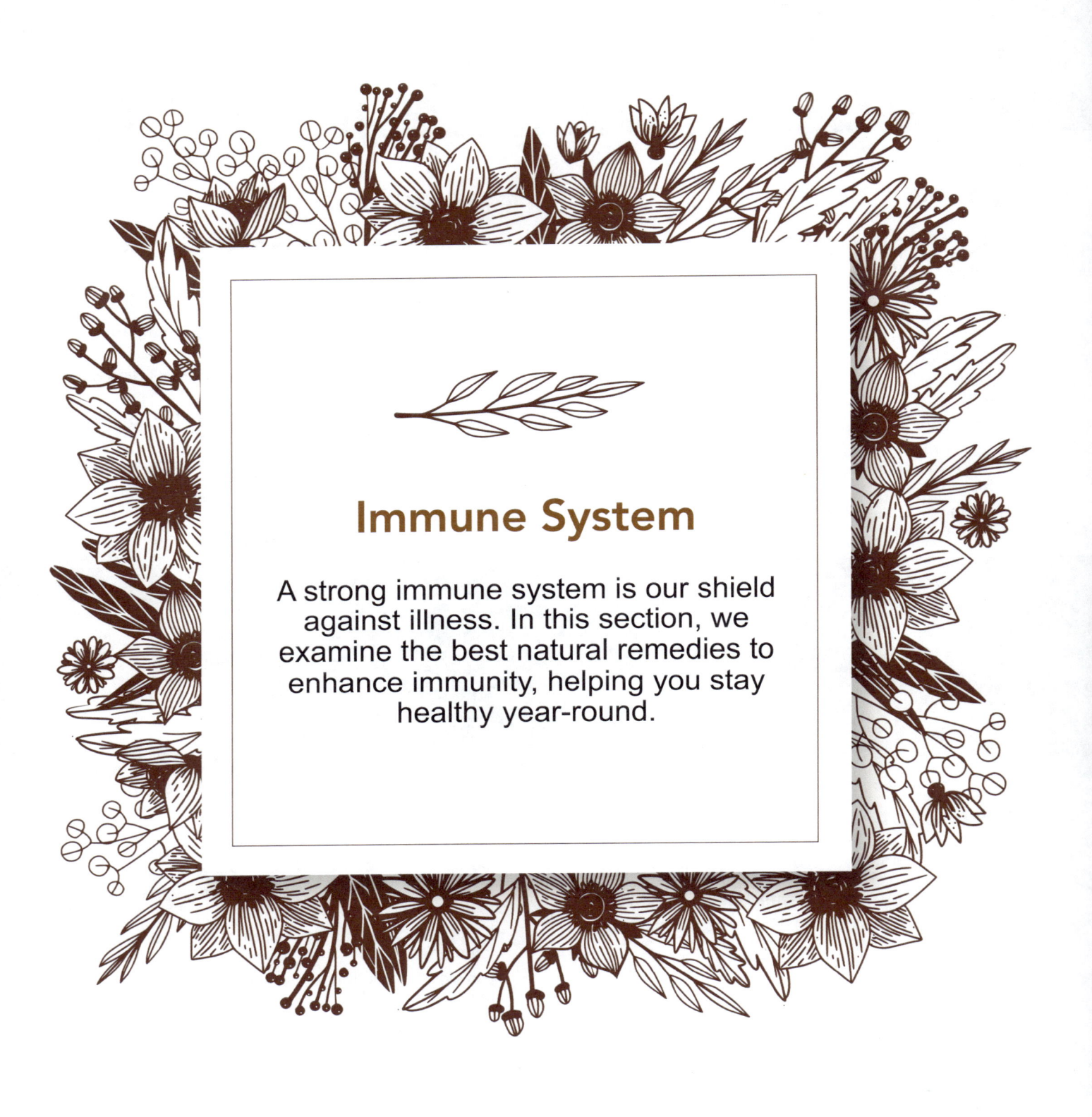

Immune System

A strong immune system is our shield against illness. In this section, we examine the best natural remedies to enhance immunity, helping you stay healthy year-round.

Healing Penicillin Soup for Cold and Flu

Penicillin Soup is a healing, traditional remedy believed to help fight off colds and flu. It's said to boost the immune system, reduce inflammation, and aid in recovery. While the name might suggest it contains actual penicillin, it typically refers to a nourishing, antimicrobial broth made with a variety of herbs and natural ingredients.

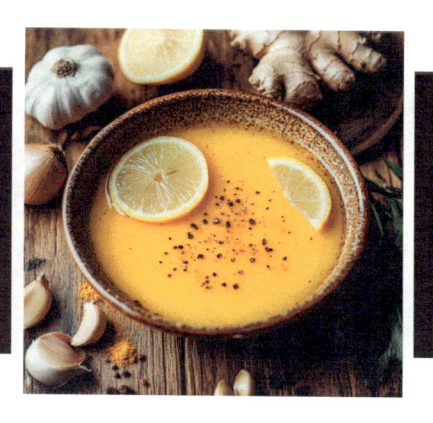

Ingredients:

- Garlic (3-4 cloves, crushed): Known for its natural antibacterial and antiviral properties, garlic is a powerful immune booster.
- Onion (1 medium, chopped): helps reduce inflammation and fight infections.
- Ginger (1 tbsp, grated): Known for its anti-inflammatory and antimicrobial properties.
- Lemon (juice of 1 lemon): Boosts vitamin C intake and supports detoxification.
- Hot Water (4 cups): Acts as the base of the soup.
- Turmeric (1 tbsp): Contains curcumin, known for its anti-inflammatory properties.
- Honey (1 tbsp): Adds sweetness and has natural antibacterial properties.

Instructions:

1. Combine all ingredients in a large pot.
2. Add water and bring to a boil, then reduce the heat and simmer for 15-20 minutes.
3. Strain the soup to remove the solid ingredients.
4. Pour the broth into a mug or bowl and enjoy while warm.

- Drink 1-2 cups of this soup daily, especially when feeling run down or fighting off illness.
- Refrigerate any leftovers for up to 2 days and reheat before consuming.

Immune-Boosting Echinacea & Astragalus Tincture

This powerful tincture combines Echinacea and Astragalus, two renowned herbs for strengthening the immune system and fighting off infections. Echinacea has long been celebrated for its ability to stimulate immune function, while Astragalus is known for its adaptogenic properties, helping the body adapt to stress and boosting overall vitality.

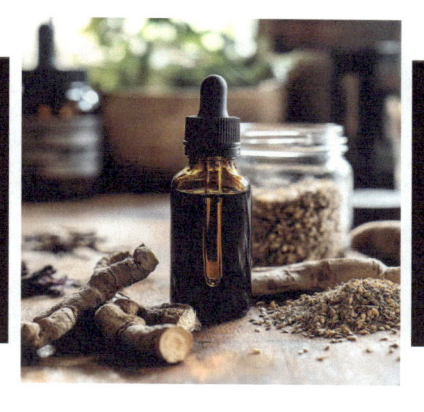

Ingredients:

- Echinacea Root (1 tablespoon, dried): A potent herb that boosts the immune system, helping to fight infections and reduce the severity of colds.
- Astragalus Root (1 tablespoon, dried): Known for its adaptogenic properties, Astragalus strengthens the body's defense mechanisms and promotes overall vitality.
- Vegetable Glycerin (or Apple Cider Vinegar, 1 cup): A gentle, alcohol-free base that extracts the herbal properties without harsh chemicals, perfect for a non-alcoholic tincture.
- Filtered Water (1/4 cup): To help with the dilution and extraction process.

Instructions:

1. Place the dried Echinacea and Astragalus root in a clean glass jar.
2. Pour the vegetable glycerin (or apple cider vinegar) over the herbs until they are fully covered.
3. Seal the jar and place it in a cool, dark area for 2-4 weeks. Shake the jar daily to ensure proper extraction.
4. After the extraction period, strain the herbs using cheesecloth or a fine mesh strainer into a clean bottle or jar.

- Take 1-2 dropperfuls in water, 1-3 times per day, particularly when you need immune support or during cold and flu season.
- Store in a cool, dark place for up to one year.

Natural Immune Support Tea

This tea can be consumed 1-3 times a day, especially when feeling the onset of cold symptoms or in situations where immune support is needed, like travel. Some recipes include variations like elderberries, rose hips, or ginger for additional immune-boosting properties, but this basic blend is simple and effective for regular use.

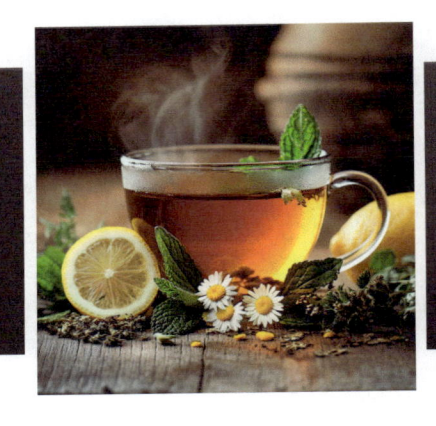

Ingredients:

- Dried nettle leaves: Rich in vitamins and minerals to support immunity.
- Dried chamomile: Provides calming effects, helping with relaxation and
- immune support.
- Fresh or dried mint: Opens sinuses and calms digestion, supporting overall respiratory health.
- Lemon juice: Adds vitamin C for an immune boost.

Instructions:

1. Use 1 tablespoon of the herbal blend per 1 cup of boiling water.
2. Let steep for about 7 minutes to extract the benefits of the herbs.
3. After steeping, add a squeeze of fresh lemon juice to enhance flavor and immunity.
- Drink 1-3 times a day, especially when feeling the onset of cold symptoms or needing immune support.
- Store in an airtight container in a cool, dry place for up to 6 months.

Anti-Inflammatory Ginger & Turmeric Root Tea

This blend is often cited for boosting immune function, reducing joint pain, and even supporting digestion due to the ginger and turmeric combination. Ginger and turmeric together also offer antioxidants, helping the body combat oxidative stress and inflammation from daily wear and tear

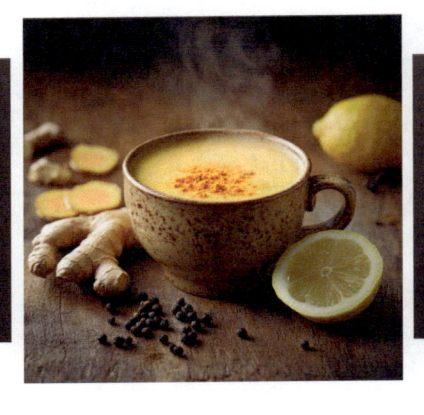

Ingredients:

- Fresh ginger root (about 1 inch, grated)
- Fresh turmeric root (1-2 inches, grated) or 1/2 teaspoon ground turmeric
- A pinch of freshly ground black pepper (enhances curcumin absorption)
- Optional: a touch of honey for sweetness and a slice of lemon for flavor

Instructions:

1. Bring 1-2 cups of water to a boil.
2. Add the grated ginger and turmeric, then reduce the heat and let it simmer for 5-10 minutes.
3. Stir in black pepper, cover, and steep for another 5 minutes to lock in the essential oils.
4. Strain and add honey or lemon to taste.
- Drink once daily, especially in the morning or evening, to support inflammation reduction.
- tore in an airtight container in a cool, dry place for up to 3 months.

Soothing Golden Turmeric & Ginger Salve

This golden salve blends turmeric and ginger to reduce pain and inflammation, making it ideal for sore muscles, joint pain, or skin irritations. Regular use enhances its effectiveness, but consult a healthcare provider if you have any health conditions.

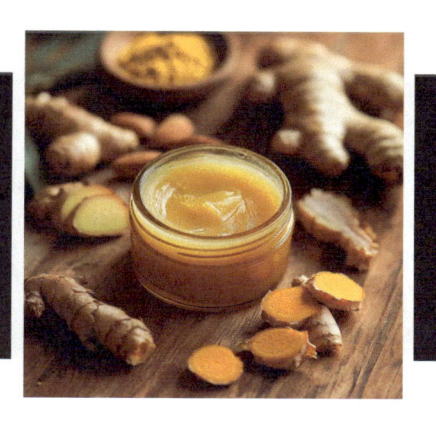

Ingredients:

- Turmeric root or turmeric powder (known for its potent anti-inflammatory properties)
- Fresh ginger root (offers additional anti-inflammatory benefits and aids in circulation)
- Beeswax (creates a stable, soothing base for the salve)
- Carrier oils (such as coconut or olive oil, to facilitate the infusion)
- Optional essential oils (e.g., lavender or frankincense for added healing properties)

Instructions:

1. Infuse the oils: Place turmeric and ginger in a carrier oil and heat gently for 1-2 hours, or let it steep in a cool place for 2 weeks.
2. Strain the infused oil using a fine mesh sieve or cheesecloth.
3. Melt beeswax in a double boiler, and add the strained oil. Stir to combine.
4. Add essential oils (optional) and stir.
5. Pour into containers: Once the mixture cools, pour it into sterilized tins or jars. Let it set before using.
- Apply a small amount of salve to sore muscles, joints, or irritated skin as needed.
- Store in a cool, dry place for up to 6 months.

Homemade Cinchona Quinine Tonic

Homemade quinine is made by extracting the potent properties from cinchona bark. It has been traditionally used to treat malaria but should be used cautiously due to its strong effects. Always consult a healthcare provider before use.

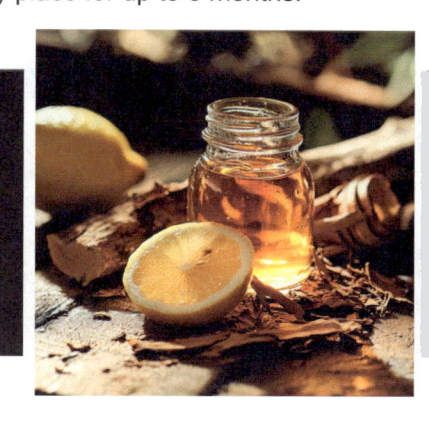

Ingredients:

- Cinchona bark (available in dried form from herb shops or online)
- Water
- Optional flavoring agents like lemon or honey (for taste)

Instructions:

1. Boil the Cinchona Bark: Start by simmering around 1 tablespoon of dried cinchona bark in about 2 cups of water for 20-30 minutes. This will extract the quinine alkaloids into the water.
2. Strain the Liquid: After boiling, strain the liquid through a fine sieve or cheesecloth to remove the bark.
3. Optional Flavoring: If desired, add honey, lemon, or other flavoring agents to help mask the bitterness of the quinine.
4. Store and Use: Store the liquid in a sealed container in the refrigerator. Use sparingly, as quinine is potent. It can be consumed as a tonic or diluted in water.
- Start with a teaspoon of tonic daily, gradually increasing the dose if needed. Dilute in water if necessary.
- Store in the refrigerator for up to 2 weeks.

Nutrient-Dense Herbal Vitamin Snack Bars

These vitamin bars are nutrient-dense snacks designed to provide natural sources of vitamins and minerals, giving a boost to your day with wholesome, energizing ingredients. These bars can be adapted to include herbs that support various health needs, from energy to immunity. Enjoy one bar as a mid-morning or afternoon snack to support energy and immune health naturally.

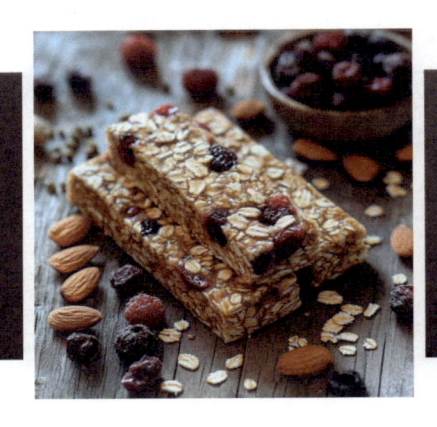

Ingredients:

- Rolled Oats: Provides fiber, B vitamins, and a hearty base for the bars.
- Honey: Adds natural sweetness and has antimicrobial properties.
- Almonds: High in vitamin E and healthy fats to support skin and immune health.
- Dried Berries (such as blueberries or goji berries): Rich in antioxidants and Vitamin C.
- Ashwagandha Powder: An adaptogen that helps the body manage stress.
- Maca Powder: Rich in iron, vitamin C, and beneficial plant compounds that support energy and mood.
- Coconut Oil: Binds ingredients together and provides healthy fats.

Instructions:

1. In a large mixing bowl, combine 1 cup of rolled oats, ¼ cup of honey, ½ cup of chopped almonds, and ¼ cup of dried berries.
2. Add 1 teaspoon of ashwagandha powder and 1 teaspoon of maca powder to the mix.
3. Melt 2 tablespoons of coconut oil and add it to the bowl, stirring thoroughly until all ingredients are well combined.
4. Press the mixture firmly into a lined 8x8-inch pan, flattening it evenly.
5. Refrigerate for 1-2 hours, then cut into bars.
6. Enjoy one bar as a mid-morning or afternoon snack to support energy and immune health.
7. Store in an airtight container in the refrigerator for up to 1 week.

Detoxifying Lymphatic Cleanser Tonic

A lymphatic cleanser can support the body's natural detox process and promote circulation in the lymphatic system, helping remove waste and toxins. This simple tonic combines ingredients that are known to stimulate lymph flow and aid digestion, supporting the body's overall well-being.

Ingredients:

- Dandelion Root: Known for its detoxifying effects, dandelion root helps stimulate the liver and kidneys, supporting waste removal.
- Burdock Root: A traditional lymphatic herb, burdock root aids in flushing out toxins and improving skin health.
- Ginger Root: Adds warmth, stimulates circulation, and helps reduce inflammation.
- Lemon Juice: High in Vitamin C, it supports immune health and acts as a natural cleanser.
- Raw Apple Cider Vinegar: Aids in digestion and has natural cleansing properties.

Instructions:

1. Combine 1 tablespoon of dandelion root, 1 tablespoon of burdock root, and 1 teaspoon of freshly grated ginger in 2 cups of water. Bring to a gentle boil, then reduce to simmer for about 10–15 minutes.
2. Strain the mixture into a cup and add the juice of half a lemon and 1–2 teaspoons of raw apple cider vinegar.
3. Stir well and enjoy warm.
- Drink this tonic once daily in the morning to encourage lymphatic flow and help the body cleanse naturally. For best results, take consistently for a week and pause if you experience any digestive discomfort.

Antiviral Mushroom Extract for Immune Support

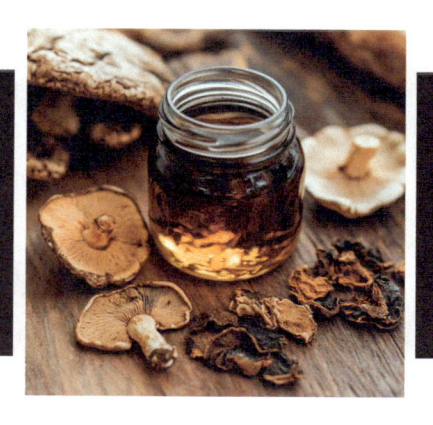

This extract blend focuses on fighting viral infections by using medicinal mushrooms known for their antiviral properties. Mushrooms like reishi, turkey tail, and chaga have been shown to contain compounds that support the body's defense mechanisms specifically against viral activity.

Ingredients:

- Reishi Mushroom: Contains triterpenes with antiviral properties that may inhibit viral replication.
- Turkey Tail Mushroom: High in polysaccharides, particularly polysaccharide-K (PSK), which has demonstrated antiviral effects and immune support.
- Shiitake Mushroom: Rich in lentinan, a beta-glucan known to help the body fight viral infections.
- Chaga Mushroom: Known for its potent antioxidants, chaga supports the body's natural defense against viruses and helps reduce inflammation.

Instructions:

1. Add 1 tablespoon each of dried reishi, turkey tail, shiitake, and chaga mushrooms to 3 cups of water in a saucepan.
2. Bring to a gentle boil, then reduce to a simmer, letting the mixture steep for 45 minutes to an hour until it reduces by half.
3. Strain the liquid into a clean jar and let it cool.
- Take 1–2 tablespoons of this extract up to twice daily, either on its own or in a warm beverage, to support your body's response to viral infections.
- Use consistently over a week or two for best results, but pause if you experience any discomfort. If you have an underlying health condition or are taking medication, consult a healthcare provider before use.

Natural Butterfly Pea Tea for Immune Support

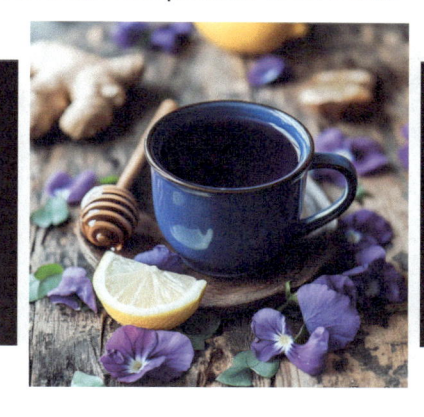

This natural remedy combines potent herbs known for their antibiotic and antimicrobial properties to support the body's fight against infections. These herbs have been traditionally used to help combat bacterial infections and enhance immune defense, making them a natural alternative to conventional antibiotics in some cases.

Ingredients:

- Butterfly Pea Flowers: Packed with antioxidants and anthocyanins to help reduce inflammation.
- Ginger: Adds anti-inflammatory properties and aids in digestion.
- Lemon: High in Vitamin C, supports immune health, and enhances the tea's color and flavor.
- Honey: Offers antimicrobial benefits and adds natural sweetness.

Instructions:

1. Boil a cup of water and add 1-2 teaspoons of butterfly pea flowers and a few slices of fresh ginger.
2. Let steep for 5-7 minutes, then strain the tea into a cup.
3. Add a squeeze of lemon juice (the tea will turn a vibrant blue-purple) and honey to taste, stirring well.
- Drink 1-2 cups daily to support inflammation reduction and boost antioxidant intake.
- This tea is especially soothing in the morning or evening. Regular use may enhance its benefits; however, consult a healthcare provider if you have specific health conditions.

Immune Boosting White Cell Juice

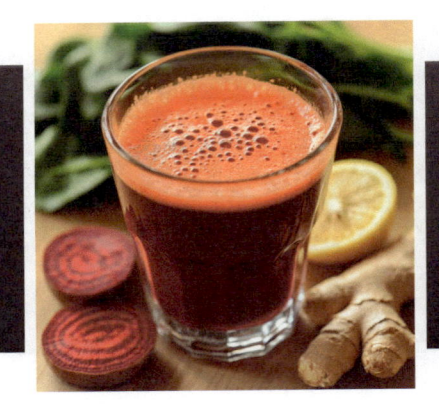

This Juice is designed to support and enhance your immune system, particularly by helping to boost white blood cells, which play a key role in fighting infections. To naturally stimulate the production of white blood cells, focus on ingredients that are rich in antioxidants, vitamins, and minerals, especially Vitamin C, Zinc, and other immune-boosting nutrients.

Ingredients:

- Carrot: High in Vitamin A and antioxidants, carrots help improve immune function.
- Lemon or Orange : Rich in Vitamin C, which is vital for the production of white blood cells and supports overall immune health.
- Spinach: A source of folate and Vitamin C, which can help boost immune cell production.
- Ginger: Contains bioactive compounds like gingerol, which have anti-inflammatory and antioxidant properties, supporting immune responses.
- Beetroot: High in antioxidants, beets help boost blood health and improve circulation, which is essential for immune function.

Instructions:

1. Start by washing all the ingredients thoroughly. Cut the carrots, beetroot, and orange into smaller pieces for easy juicing.
2. Juice the carrots, beetroot, spinach, ginger, lemon, and orange together.
3. Serve: Stir the juice and serve fresh. You can add a bit of honey for sweetness.
- Drink daily to help support immune health and boost white blood cell production.
- Store in an airtight container in the refrigerator for up to 2 days.

Nature's Antibiotic Capsules

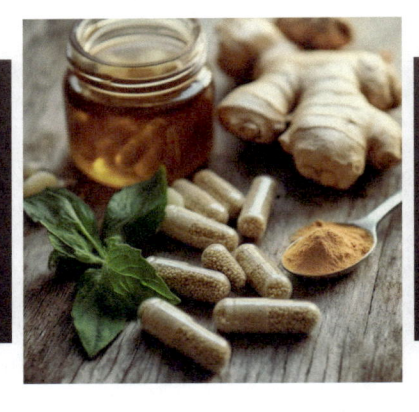

Herbal antibiotic capsules are an excellent natural remedy to support your immune system and help combat bacterial infections. These capsules contain a combination of powerful herbs known for their antibacterial properties, making them an effective and convenient alternative to traditional antibiotics.

Ingredients:

- Garlic: Contains allicin, a compound with strong antibacterial properties that helps combat various infections.
- Oregano: Oregano oil has carvacrol, a potent antimicrobial compound that fights bacterial infections, especially in the respiratory tract.
- Ginger: Known for its ability to fight inflammation and infection, ginger is also a natural antibacterial and immune booster.
- Honey: Especially Manuka honey, which is rich in antibacterial properties, it's useful for treating wounds and digestive infections.

Instructions:

1. Prepare the Ingredients: You'll need dried garlic powder, ginger powder, and oregano oil or extract. Use Manuka honey powder (if available) or use raw honey for internal consumption.
2. Fill the Capsules: Use empty gelatin or vegetarian capsules. A capsule filling machine will help you make larger batches.
3. Take one capsule daily for general immune support, or two to three capsules when dealing with an infection.
4. Capsules can be taken with or without food, alongside plenty of water for better absorption.

Amish Fire Cider

This is a traditional, homemade tonic made with a mix of apple cider vinegar, spices, and other herbs. It's known for its ability to support the immune system, improve digestion, and promote overall health. Often used as a natural remedy during cold and flu season, it's packed with anti-inflammatory, antimicrobial, and immune-boosting ingredients.

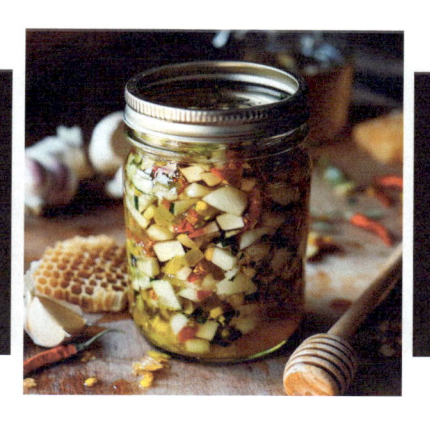

Ingredients:

- Apple Cider Vinegar: Helps balance the body's pH and supports digestion.
- Garlic: A powerful antimicrobial that boosts immunity.
- Ginger: Provides anti-inflammatory benefits and aids digestion.
- Horseradish: Supports respiratory health and helps clear congestion.
- Chili Peppers: Contain capsaicin, which stimulates circulation and supports the immune system.
- Honey: Adds natural sweetness and has soothing, antimicrobial properties.

Instructions:

1. Chop the garlic, ginger, horseradish, and chili peppers, then add them to a quart-sized jar, filling it halfway.
2. Pour apple cider vinegar over the ingredients, covering them completely.
3. Seal the jar tightly, shake to mix, and store in a cool, dark place for 2-3 weeks, shaking daily.
4. After 2-3 weeks, strain the mixture through a fine mesh strainer or cheesecloth.
5. Add honey to taste, stirring until dissolved.
- Take 1-2 tablespoons daily for general immune support or 1 tablespoon every 4-6 hours when feeling unwell. If the taste is too strong, dilute with water, juice, or tea.

Blue Tea Bliss

Blue tea, made from butterfly pea flowers, is not only beautiful but also rich in antioxidants and compounds that help combat inflammation. This soothing tea is perfect for easing inflammatory discomfort and promoting overall wellness.

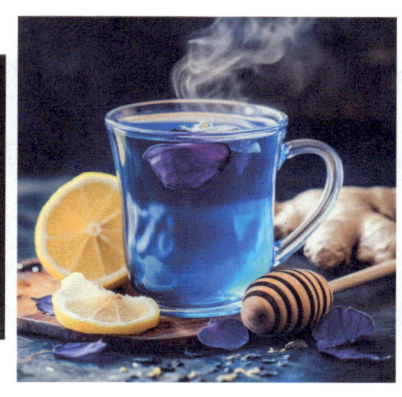

Ingredients:

- Butterfly Pea Flowers: Packed with antioxidants and anthocyanins to help reduce inflammation.
- Ginger: Adds anti-inflammatory properties and aids in digestion.
- Lemon: High in Vitamin C, supports immune health, and enhances the tea's color and flavor.
- Honey: Offers antimicrobial benefits and adds natural sweetness.

Instructions:

1. Boil a cup of water and add 1-2 teaspoons of butterfly pea flowers and a few slices of fresh ginger.
2. Let steep for 5-7 minutes, then strain the tea into a cup.
3. Add a squeeze of lemon juice (the tea will turn a vibrant blue-purple) and honey to taste, stirring well.
- Drink 1-2 cups daily to support inflammation reduction and boost antioxidant intake. This tea is especially soothing in the morning or evening. Regular use may enhance its benefits; however, consult a healthcare provider if you have specific health conditions.

Fungal Fighter Cream

This homemade herbal cream combines antifungal and soothing ingredients traditionally used to treat nail fungus. The herbs used in this remedy have powerful antimicrobial properties, which can help fight the fungal infection while promoting healing.

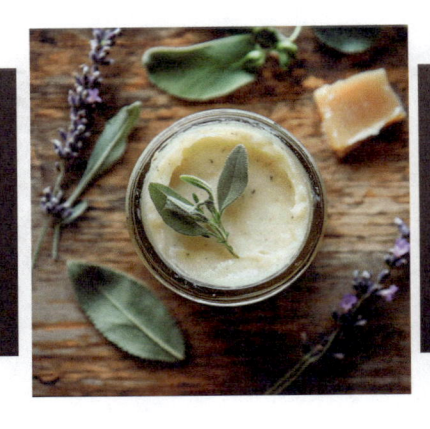

Ingredients:

- Tea Tree Oil: Known for its potent antifungal and antibacterial properties, tea tree oil is a popular remedy for fungal infections.
- Oregano Oil: Contains carvacrol, which has antifungal effects, especially useful for treating nail fungus.
- Coconut Oil: A natural moisturizer, coconut oil also has antifungal properties, which can help soothe the skin around the infected nail.
- Lavender Oil: Known for its calming properties, lavender oil also has mild antifungal effects, making it beneficial in soothing the skin during treatment.
- Beeswax: Acts as a natural thickener to help create a cream-like consistency, while also offering antibacterial properties.

Instructions:

1. In a double boiler, melt 1 tablespoon of beeswax along with 2 tablespoons of coconut oil until fully liquefied.
2. Once the mixture is melted, remove from heat and add 10 drops of tea tree oil, 5 drops of oregano oil, and 5 drops of lavender oil. Stir well to combine.
3. Allow the mixture to cool and solidify into a cream-like consistency.
4. Transfer the cream into a small glass jar for storage.
- Apply the herbal cream directly to the affected nail and surrounding skin twice daily.

Fungal Relief Salve

This antifungal salve uses a blend of soothing oils and herbs to help combat fungal infections, particularly those affecting the nails or skin. Lavender and eucalyptus essential oils work alongside calendula and beeswax to create a healing, moisturizing salve that can help reduce fungal growth and promote skin recovery.

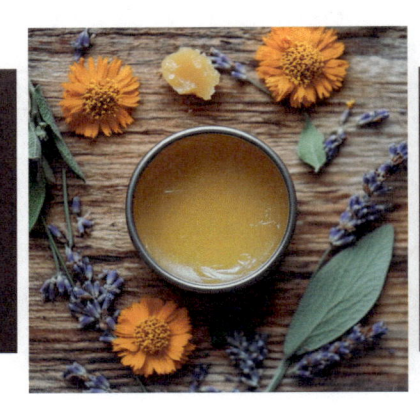

Ingredients:

- Olive Oil: A mild carrier oil with natural antifungal properties.
- Lavender Essential Oil: Known for its antifungal, soothing, and healing qualities.
- Eucalyptus Oil: Contains antifungal compounds that help fight fungal infections.
- Calendula Flowers: Promotes healing and reduces inflammation, beneficial for irritated or infected skin.
- Beeswax: Solidifies the salve, creating a spreadable consistency.

Instructions:

1. Infuse Calendula: Place dried calendula flowers in olive oil and let it steep for 1-2 weeks, shaking occasionally to ensure the oil absorbs the medicinal properties.
2. Prepare the Salve Base: In a double boiler, melt beeswax. Once melted, mix in the calendula-infused olive oil.
3. Add Essential Oils: Once the beeswax and oil mixture is blended and slightly cooled, add lavender and eucalyptus essential oils for their antifungal properties.
4. Pour and Set: Pour the mixture into a small jar or tin and let it cool and solidify.
- Apply to affected areas 2-3 times daily. This salve can be used on toenail fungus, athlete's foot, or other fungal skin infections. For best results, continue use until the infection is completely healed. If irritation occurs, discontinue use and consult a healthcare provider.

Natural Anti Wart Spray

This spray provides a natural way to treat warts by mimicking the freezing method used in conventional over-the-counter wart treatments. It utilizes simple, effective ingredients known for their ability to freeze and eliminate warts over time, without harsh chemicals.

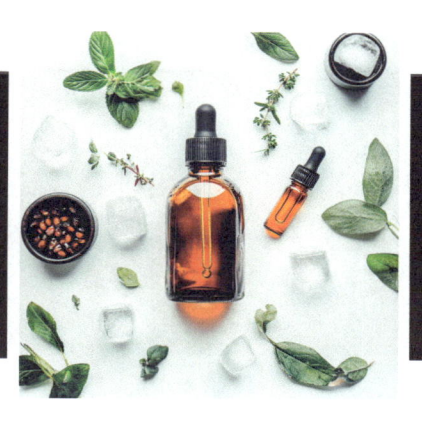

Ingredients:

- Witch Hazel: An astringent that helps soothe the skin and reduce inflammation.
- Apple Cider Vinegar: Known for its ability to break down wart tissue over time.
- Tea Tree Oil: Antifungal and antiviral properties make it a good remedy for warts.
- Ice: Freezing the wart is the key to causing it to shrink and fall off.

Instructions:

1. Mix 2 tablespoons of apple cider vinegar, 1 tablespoon of witch hazel, and 10 drops of tea tree oil in a spray bottle.
2. Wrap a small piece of ice in a cloth or gauze, applying it directly to the wart for 10-15 minutes.
3. Spray the wart with the apple cider vinegar mixture after freezing. Allow it to air dry.
- Apply the spray to the wart twice a day, and repeat the freezing process with ice for 10-15 minutes daily. The wart should begin to shrink and eventually fall off after several treatments, typically within 1-2 weeks. If discomfort or irritation occurs, discontinue use and consult a healthcare provider.

Candida Relief Ointment

This natural ointment targets Candida overgrowth on the skin, helping to soothe discomfort while gently cleansing and protecting the affected area. The ingredients in this blend have natural antifungal, antibacterial, and skin-soothing properties.

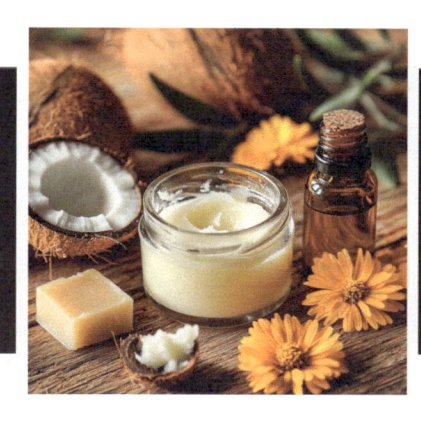

Ingredients:

- Coconut Oil: Naturally antifungal, coconut oil can help disrupt the cell walls of Candida.
- Tea Tree Oil: Known for its strong antifungal and antibacterial effects, especially helpful in combating Candida on the skin.
- Calendula Oil: Adds soothing, anti-inflammatory benefits to reduce irritation and redness.
- Beeswax: Acts as a natural preservative and creates a protective barrier to prevent moisture from aggravating the infection.

Instructions:

1. In a double boiler, melt 2 tablespoons of coconut oil and 1 tablespoon of beeswax until smooth.
2. Remove from heat, then add 10 drops of tea tree oil and 1 tablespoon of calendula oil. Stir well.
3. Pour the mixture into a small glass container and let it cool until it solidifies.
- Apply a thin layer of this ointment to affected areas once or twice daily after gently cleansing and drying the skin. Use consistently to support healing. Discontinue use if irritation occurs, and consult a healthcare provider for persistent or severe symptoms.
- Store in a cool, dry place, and use within a month for maximum freshness.

Viral Relief Oil

This soothing oil blend is designed to relieve irritation, reduce inflammation, and help address viral activity associated with herpes sores and shingles. The ingredients used have natural antiviral, anti-inflammatory, and skin-soothing properties.

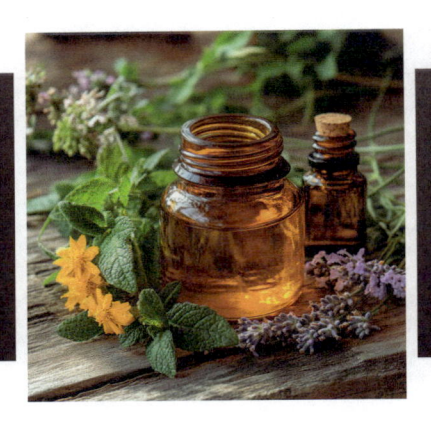

Ingredients:

- St. John's Wort Oil: Known for its antiviral and nerve-soothing properties, making it effective for shingles and herpes.
- Lemon Balm Oil: A powerful antiviral that has shown effectiveness against the herpes simplex virus.
- Tea Tree Oil: Contains antiviral and antiseptic properties, ideal for cleansing and soothing sores.
- Lavender Oil: Calms irritation and inflammation while also supporting the skin's healing process.

Instructions:

1. Combine Oils: In a small glass jar, mix 1 tablespoon of St. John's Wort oil, 1 tablespoon of lemon balm oil, 5 drops of tea tree oil, and 5 drops of lavender oil.
2. Blend and Store: Stir the mixture well. Seal the jar tightly and store it in a cool, dark place.
- Apply a small amount of the oil blend directly to affected areas up to 3 times daily, using a cotton swab to avoid contamination. For sensitive skin, test a small patch first or dilute further with a neutral carrier oil. Avoid using on broken skin or open sores.
- Store in a cool, dry place, and use within three months for optimal freshness.

Herpes Comfort Balm

This herbal balm is designed to help alleviate the discomfort and inflammation associated with herpes sores. With antiviral and calming properties, this balm aims to provide relief while promoting skin healing.

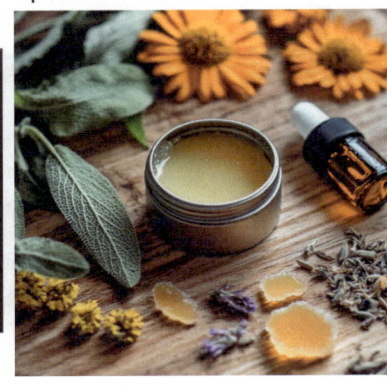

Ingredients:

- Lemon Balm: Known for its antiviral effects, especially against the herpes simplex virus.
- Calendula: Helps soothe inflamed skin and supports healing.
- Coconut Oil: Antiviral and moisturizing, helping to prevent cracking and irritation.
- Beeswax: Acts as a base to create the balm's consistency and provides a protective layer.
- Tea Tree Oil: Has potent antiviral and antimicrobial properties to fight infection.

Instructions:

1. In a double boiler, melt 1/4 cup of coconut oil with 2 tablespoons of beeswax until fully combined.
2. Add 1 tablespoon of dried lemon balm and calendula flowers; let them infuse over low heat for 10–15 minutes.
3. Strain out the herbs, then stir in 5–10 drops of tea tree oil.
4. Pour the mixture into a small container and allow it to solidify.
- Apply a small amount directly to the affected area up to twice daily. Store the balm in a cool, dry place, and use within three months. If you experience irritation, discontinue use, and consult a healthcare provider.

Heavy Metal Cleanse Powder

This natural detox blend supports the body in eliminating heavy metals that can accumulate due to environmental factors. Key ingredients help to bind with and clear heavy metals, while promoting liver and kidney health to optimize natural detoxification processes.

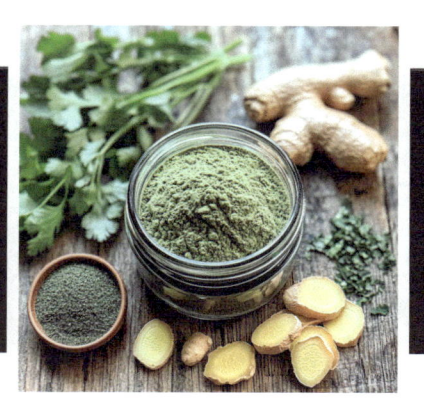

Ingredients:

- Cilantro: Known for its ability to bind heavy metals, helping to facilitate their removal from tissues.
- Chlorella: A green algae high in chlorophyll that binds to heavy metals, supporting detox through the digestive system.
- Milk Thistle: Supports liver health and function, aiding the body's natural detoxification.
- Ginger Root: Stimulates digestion and supports circulation, aiding in the transport and removal of toxins.

Instructions:

1. Combine 1 tablespoon of dried cilantro and 1 teaspoon each of chlorella powder, dried milk thistle, and dried ginger root in a small bowl.
2. Blend these ingredients into a fine powder.
3. Store in an airtight container in a cool, dark place.
- Take 1/2 teaspoon of this mixture daily, either in a glass of water, smoothie, or juice. For best results, use consistently for one to two weeks, then pause to avoid overloading the body. Consult a healthcare provider before starting, especially if you have pre-existing conditions.

Immune Soothing Mushroom Tincture

These mushroom drops help regulate an overactive immune response, particularly for conditions where calming the immune system is beneficial. Certain medicinal mushrooms contain compounds that can balance immune activity, reducing inflammation and supporting overall wellness.

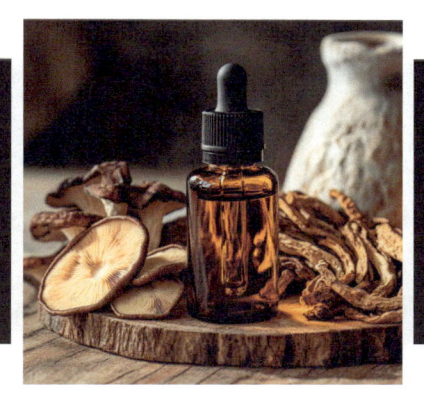

Ingredients:

- Reishi Mushroom: Contains triterpenes that may help modulate immune function, easing an overactive response.
- Cordyceps Mushroom: Known for its adaptogenic properties, supporting balanced immune responses and reducing stress on the immune system.
- Turkey Tail Mushroom: Contains polysaccharides that support immune health without overstimulation.
- Astragalus Root: Often used for immune regulation, helping to calm excessive immune responses.

Instructions:

1. Place 1 tablespoon each of dried reishi, cordyceps, and turkey tail mushrooms, along with astragalus root, into a glass jar.
2. Cover with high-proof alcohol, filling the jar to just above the herbs.
3. Seal and let sit for 4–6 weeks, shaking gently every few days.
4. Strain the liquid into a dropper bottle.
- Take 1–2 droppers daily, either on its own or added to a beverage. Consistent use over several weeks can help regulate immune function.
- Store in a cool, dark place for up to a year.

Elderberry Immunity Boost Syrup

This elderberry syrup is a powerful immune booster, known for its ability to help fight off cold and flu viruses. Elderberries are rich in antioxidants, vitamins, and flavonoids, which help strengthen the immune system and combat infections.

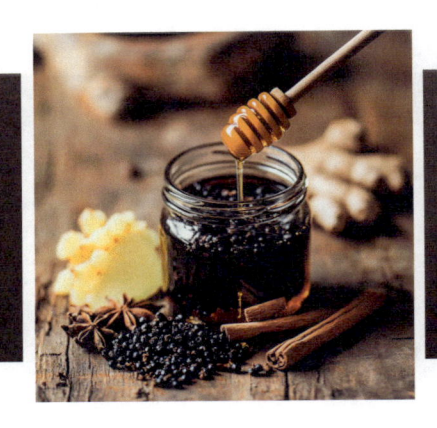

Ingredients:

- Elderberries (1 cup, dried or fresh): Known for their antiviral properties, elderberries are packed with antioxidants, vitamin C, and other immune-boosting compounds.
- Honey (1/2 cup): helps soothe the throat and further supports the immune system.
- Cinnamon (1 stick): Known for its anti-inflammatory and antimicrobial properties, cinnamon supports immune health.
- Cloves (3-4 whole): Contain antioxidants and have been traditionally used for their antimicrobial effects.
- Ginger (1 small piece, sliced): Known for its warming and anti-inflammatory effects, ginger boosts circulation and helps relieve symptoms of cold & flu.
- Water (4 cups): Used as the base for the syrup.

Instructions:

1. Combine elderberries, cinnamon stick, cloves, and ginger in a pot with water.
2. Bring to a boil, then reduce to a simmer for 30-45 minutes, until the liquid reduces by half.
3. Strain out the herbs and berries, then stir in honey while the syrup is still warm.
4. Let the syrup cool completely before transferring it to a clean jar or bottle.
- Take 1-2 tablespoons daily to boost immunity, or take 1 tablespoon every few hours at the first sign of illness.
- Store in an airtight container in the refrigerator for up to 2-3 months.

Anti-Inflammatory Turmeric Milk

Golden Milk is a soothing and flavorful drink, packed with turmeric, which is well-known for its powerful anti-inflammatory properties. This warm, comforting drink is perfect for soothing joint pain, promoting digestion, and supporting overall wellness.

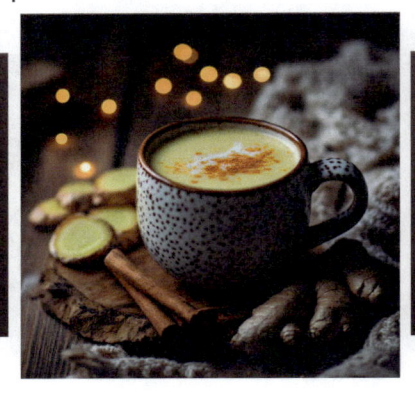

Ingredients:

- Turmeric Powder (1 teaspoon): Provides the anti-inflammatory compound curcumin.
- Milk (1 cup, dairy or plant-based): Acts as a smooth base for the drink and provides calcium.
- Black Pepper (1/4 teaspoon): Boosts curcumin absorption.
- Honey (1 teaspoon): Adds sweetness and additional anti-inflammatory benefits.
- Cinnamon (optional, 1/2 teaspoon): Offers its own anti-inflammatory properties and a warm, comforting flavor.
- Ginger (optional, 1/2 teaspoon, fresh or powdered): Known for its anti-inflammatory effects and digestive benefits.

Instructions:

1. Heat the milk gently over medium heat.
2. Add turmeric, black pepper, and cinnamon or ginger, stirring to combine.
3. Let it warm for 2-3 minutes (don't let it boil).
4. Remove from heat and stir in honey.
5. Pour into a mug and enjoy.
- Sip 1 cup daily, especially before bed, to reduce inflammation and relax.
- Drink fresh for maximum potency, or store in the fridge for up to 2 days. Reheat before consuming.

Immune-Boosting Herbal Honey

This antiviral herbal honey combines the immune-boosting properties of raw honey and powerful medicinal herbs, creating a natural remedy to support your body against infections and viruses. It is ideal for soothing sore throats, boosting immunity, and providing natural antibacterial and antiviral effects.

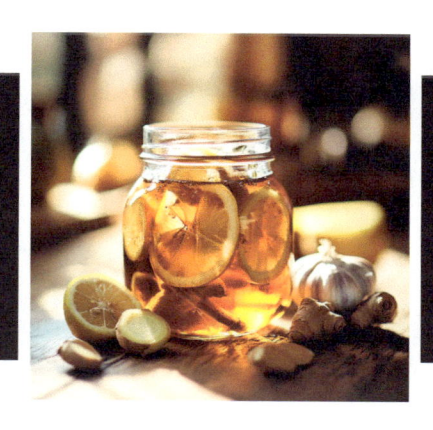

Ingredients:

- Raw Honey (1 cup): Natural antibacterial properties that help soothe sore throats and support the immune system.
- Garlic (3-4 cloves, finely chopped): Known for its antiviral and antibacterial effects.
- Echinacea Root (1 tablespoon, dried): Boosts the immune system and reduces the severity of infections.
- Ginger Root (1 tablespoon, fresh or dried): Helps fight viruses and bacteria, as well as reduces inflammation.
- Lemon (juice of 1 lemon): High in vitamin C, which supports immune function and aids in detoxification.

Instructions:

1. Combine the raw honey, chopped garlic, echinacea root, ginger, and lemon juice in a glass jar.
2. Seal the jar and let the herbs infuse in the honey for 2-3 weeks in a cool, dark place, shaking occasionally.
3. Strain the herbs out before using if desired.
- Take 1 teaspoon daily for immune support, or 1 teaspoon every 2-3 hours at the first sign of illness.
- Keep in a cool, dark place. The honey will last for several months and become more potent over time as it infuses.

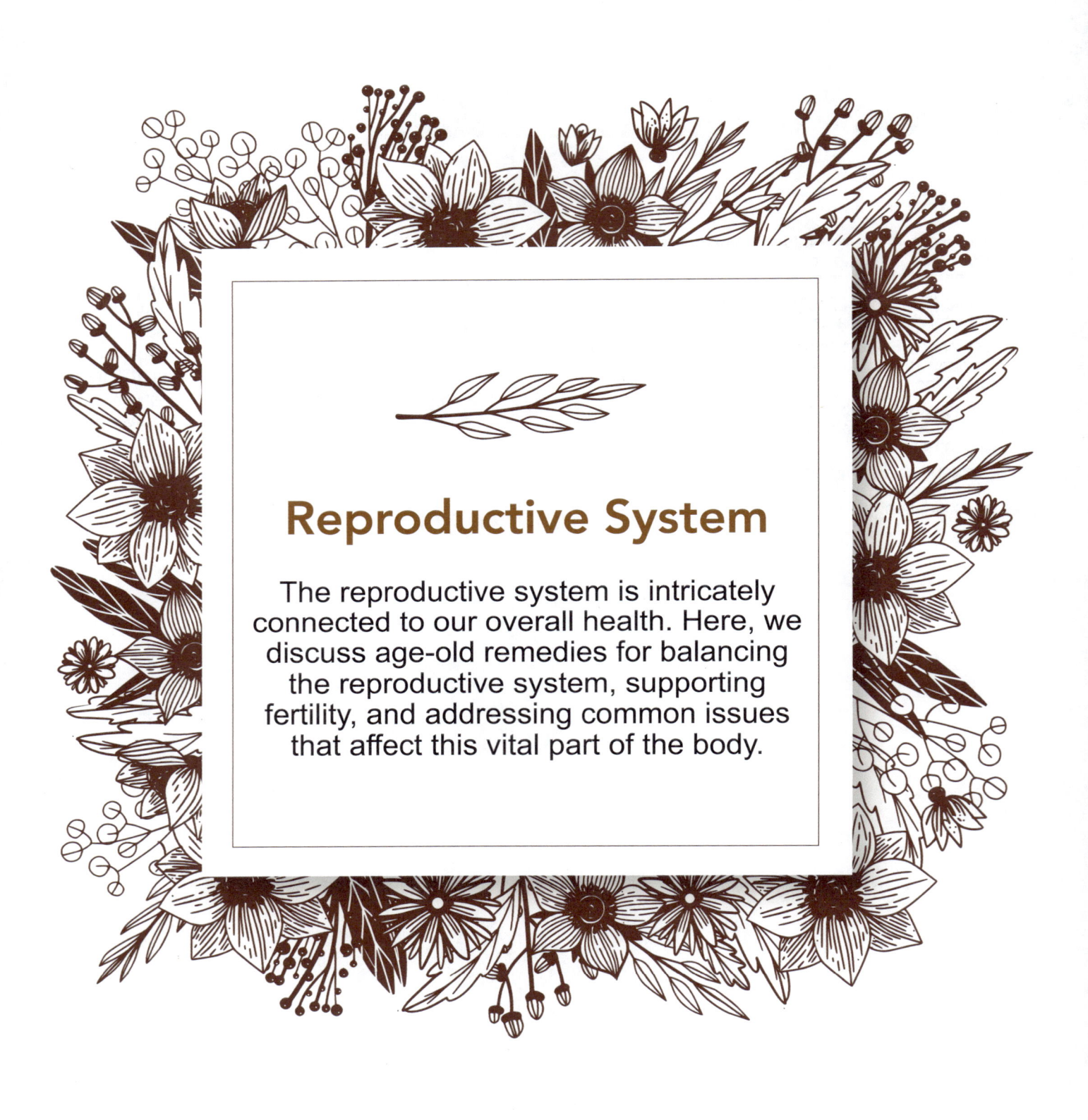

Reproductive System

The reproductive system is intricately connected to our overall health. Here, we discuss age-old remedies for balancing the reproductive system, supporting fertility, and addressing common issues that affect this vital part of the body.

Hormonal Balance Menopause Elixir

This soothing elixir is designed to alleviate common menopause symptoms, such as hot flashes, mood swings, and hormonal imbalances, using a blend of hormone-supporting herbs.

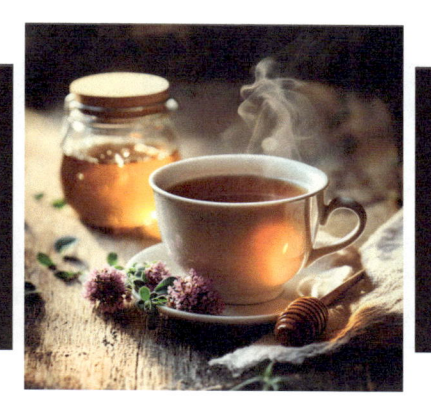

Ingredients:

- Red Clover (1 tablespoon): Rich in phytoestrogens that can help balance hormones and reduce hot flashes.
- Black Cohosh Root (1 teaspoon): Known for reducing hot flashes and night sweats.
- Dong Quai (1/2 teaspoon): Traditionally used for hormone regulation and to ease menopausal symptoms.
- Honey (1 teaspoon): Adds a touch of sweetness and soothing effects.

Instructions:

1. Combine red clover, black cohosh root, and dong quai in 1 cup of hot water.
2. Allow the mixture to steep for 10-15 minutes.
3. Strain, then stir in honey.

- Drink 1 cup daily to support symptom relief during menopause.
- Store in an airtight container in a cool, dark place for up to 1 week. Reheat before drinking, if desired.

Menstrual Relief Anise Seed Tea

This herbal tea is crafted to ease menstrual cramping and pain through the anti-inflammatory and muscle-relaxing properties of anise seed. Known for its ability to soothe the digestive system and relax muscles, this tea provides natural relief from discomfort associated with dysmenorrhea.

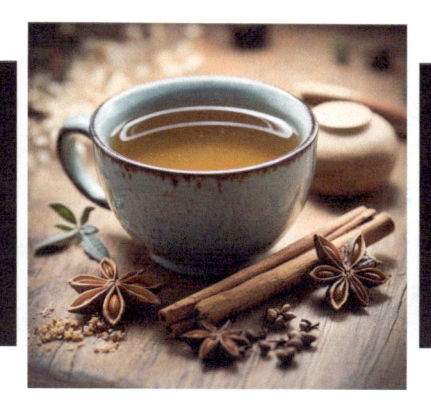

Ingredients:

- Anise Seeds (1 teaspoon): Known for their anti-inflammatory properties, anise seeds help relieve menstrual cramps and discomfort.
- Cinnamon (1/4 teaspoon): A warming spice that improves circulation and reduces pain.
- Honey (1 teaspoon): Soothes the digestive tract and adds a touch of natural sweetness.
- Water (1 cup): The base for brewing the tea.

Instructions:

1. Combine anise seeds and cinnamon in a cup of hot water.
2. Let the mixture steep for 10-15 minutes.
3. Strain, then stir in honey to sweeten.

- Drink 1 cup of tea before or during your period to help alleviate menstrual cramps and discomfort.
- Store in an airtight container in a cool, dark place for up to 1 week. Reheat before drinking if desired.

Lunar Harmony Tea

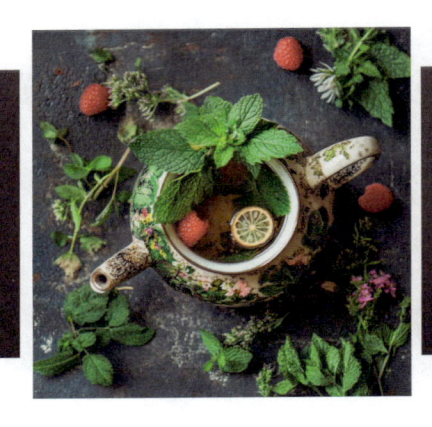

This soothing tea is designed to support the female reproductive system, particularly during menstruation. The blend of herbs works to balance hormones, relieve cramps, and ease tension, promoting a sense of calm and balance.

Ingredients:

- Red Raspberry Leaf (1 tablespoon): Known for its ability to tone the uterus and support reproductive health.
- Nettle Leaf (1 tablespoon): Provides vitamins and minerals essential for hormonal balance and supports overall health.
- Dong Quai Root (1 teaspoon): Traditionally used to balance hormones and support menstrual regularity.
- Lemon Balm (1 teaspoon): Soothes the nervous system and eases tension and stress.
- Peppermint (1/2 teaspoon): Adds a refreshing flavor and aids in relieving cramps.

Instructions:

1. Combine all herbs in a heatproof jar or teapot.
2. Pour 1 cup of hot water over the herbs and let steep for 10–15 minutes.
3. Strain and enjoy.
- Drink 1–2 cups daily, especially during menstruation or as needed for reproductive support.

Hormonal Balance & Skin Care Primrose Oil

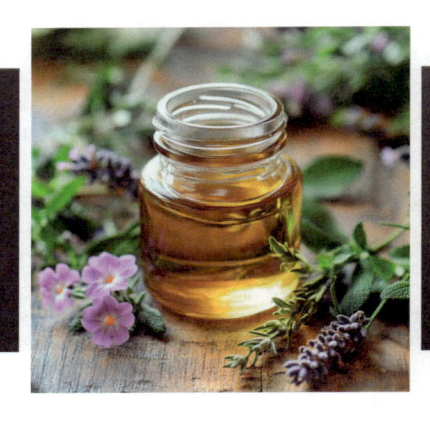

This herbal oil blend combines the benefits of natural ingredients to support hormonal balance, reduce PMS symptoms, and promote skin health. The infusion of herbs and oils works synergistically to provide relief and enhance overall well-being.

Ingredients:

- Evening Primrose Oil (2 tablespoons): Supports hormonal balance and skin health.
- Chaste Tree Berry (Vitex) (1 teaspoon, dried or powdered): Known for supporting hormone regulation, especially during PMS and menopause.
- Lavender Essential Oil (5 drops): Calms the nervous system and supports emotional balance.
- Rosehip Oil (1 tablespoon): High in vitamin C, supports skin regeneration, and helps with inflammation.
- Jojoba Oil (1 tablespoon): Acts as a base oil that helps nourish and hydrate the skin.

Instructions:

1. In a small glass jar, combine evening primrose oil, chaste tree berry, rosehip oil, and jojoba oil.
2. Add lavender essential oil and stir gently to mix.
3. Seal the jar and let the mixture sit in a cool, dark place for 1-2 weeks to infuse.
4. After the infusion period, strain the herbs out using a fine mesh sieve or cheesecloth.
5. Store the infused oil in a clean, sealed bottle or jar.
- Take 1-2 teaspoons orally for hormone balance, or massage a small amount onto the skin for nourishment and relief from PMS symptoms.
- Store in a cool, dark place for up to 6 months.

Lactation Support Herbal Tea

This herbal tea blend is designed to help support lactation by enhancing milk production in nursing mothers. With ingredients known for their galactagogue properties, it promotes healthy milk flow, balances hormones, and nourishes the body during breastfeeding.

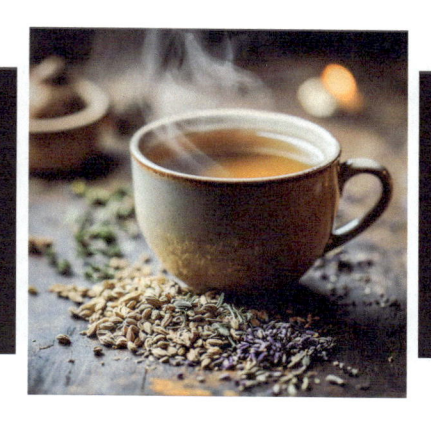

Ingredients:

- Fenugreek (1 teaspoon, seeds or powder): Fenugreek is widely used to enhance milk production and is considered one of the most effective herbs for breastfeeding mothers.
- Fennel Seeds (1 teaspoon): Fennel is another galactagogue herb known to support milk supply and improve digestion.
- Blessed Thistle (1 teaspoon): Often used alongside fenugreek, blessed thistle helps stimulate milk production and is beneficial for overall breast health.
- Water (1 cup): To brew the tea.

Instructions:

1. Add fenugreek, fennel seeds, and blessed thistle to a cup of hot water.
2. Steep for 10-15 minutes.
3. Strain out the herbs and enjoy.
- Drink 1-2 cups daily to support lactation and milk flow.
- Store any leftover tea in the fridge for up to 24 hours. Reheat as needed.

Menstrual Comfort Herb Tincture

This powerful herbal tincture combines three herbs traditionally used to address menstrual issues such as cramps, heavy bleeding, and irregular cycles. Each herb in this blend offers specific benefits for menstrual health, making it a natural and holistic remedy.

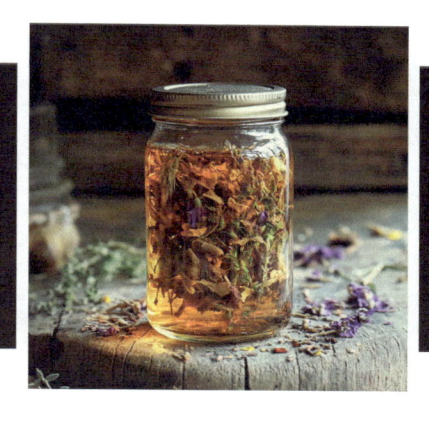

Ingredients:

- Cramp Bark (1 tablespoon, dried): Known for its ability to relieve uterine cramps and spasms.
- Red Clover (1 tablespoon, dried): Supports hormonal balance and promotes menstrual cycle regularity.
- Vegetable Glycerin (1 cup): Alcohol-free extraction medium for a gentle, sweet tincture.

Instructions:

1. Combine the Cramp Bark and Red Clover in a clean glass jar.
2. Add the vegetable glycerin, ensuring the herbs are fully submerged.
3. Seal the jar and let it sit in a cool, dark place for 2-4 weeks, shaking daily.
4. Strain the herbs using cheesecloth or a fine mesh strainer.
- Take 1-2 dropperfuls in water, once or twice a day, especially during menstruation to ease cramps.
- Store in a cool, dark place for up to one year.

Fertility Support Tonic

This fertility-boosting tonic combines nourishing herbs traditionally used to support hormonal balance, improve reproductive health, and boost fertility. Packed with nutrients and antioxidants, it helps stimulate circulation to the reproductive organs, regulate menstrual cycles, and balance hormones.

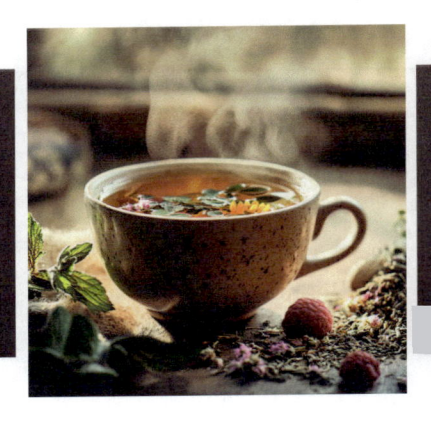

Ingredients:

- Red Clover (1 teaspoon): Known for its estrogenic properties, red clover helps balance hormone levels and improve reproductive health.
- Nettle Leaf (1 teaspoon): Rich in vitamins and minerals, nettle supports uterine health and overall fertility.
- Raspberry Leaf (1 teaspoon): Helps tone the uterus and regulate menstrual cycles.
- Honey (1 teaspoon): Naturally sweetens and adds soothing properties.
- Water (1 cup): The base for steeping the herbs.

Instructions:

1. Combine the red clover, nettle leaf, and raspberry leaf in a cup of hot water.
2. Let the mixture steep for 10-15 minutes.
3. Strain the herbs out, then stir in honey.
- Drink 1 cup of this tonic daily, especially during the first half of your menstrual cycle, to help promote fertility and balance reproductive health.
- Store the tonic in an airtight container in a cool, dark place for up to 1 week. Reheat before drinking if desired.

Nature's Fertility Aphrodisiac

This potent blend of herbs is crafted to stimulate the senses, improve libido, and support overall reproductive health. Combining aphrodisiac herbs with nourishing botanicals, this tonic can help balance hormones, improve circulation, and enhance energy.

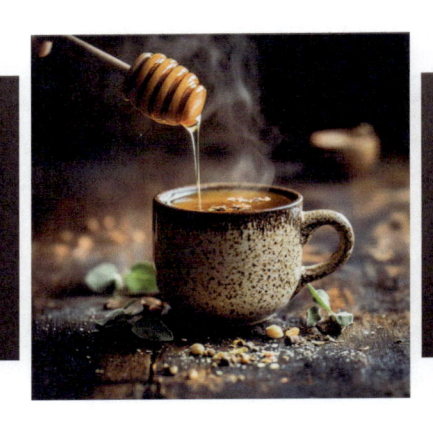

Ingredients:

- Maca Root (1 teaspoon): Known for its ability to increase libido and support hormonal balance.
- Damiana (1 teaspoon): A powerful aphrodisiac herb that supports sexual health and vitality.
- Ashwagandha (1 teaspoon): Helps reduce stress and balance hormones, promoting overall reproductive health.
- Honey (1 teaspoon): Naturally sweetens the tonic and provides energy-boosting properties.
- Water (1 cup): The base for the herbal infusion.

Instructions:

1. Combine the maca root, damiana, and ashwagandha in a cup of hot water.
2. Let steep for 10-15 minutes.
3. Strain the herbs out, then stir in honey to taste.
- Consume 1 cup of the tonic daily, ideally in the morning or before bed, to support libido and reproductive health.
- Store the tonic in an airtight container in a cool, dark place for up to 1 week. Reheat as needed.

Male Vitality Herbal Tonic

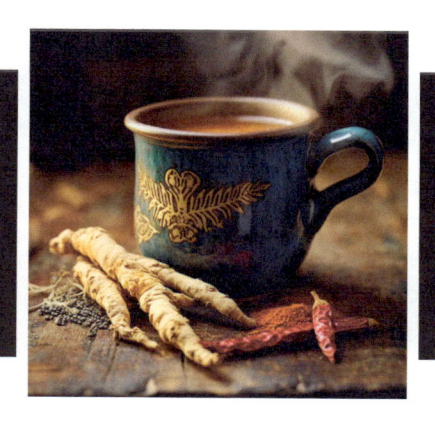

This herbal blend is crafted to support male reproductive health and enhance circulation, which may help improve erectile function. Combining traditional herbs known for their ability to boost vitality and blood flow, this tonic can be a natural aid in addressing erectile dysfunction.

Ingredients:

- Ginseng (1 teaspoon): Known for its ability to improve circulation and boost energy levels, ginseng is traditionally used to support sexual health.
- Maca Root (1 teaspoon): A popular herb used to enhance stamina and libido, maca may help balance hormone levels and improve reproductive function.
- Horny Goat Weed (1 teaspoon): This herb is traditionally used to enhance sexual health and is believed to improve blood flow to the genital area.
- Cayenne Pepper (1/4 teaspoon): Known for its ability to stimulate circulation and improve blood flow, which can help with erectile function.
- Water (1 cup): For making the infusion.

Instructions:

1. Add the ginseng, maca root, horny goat weed, and cayenne pepper to a cup of hot water.
2. Let it steep for 10-15 minutes.
3. Strain the herbs out and enjoy the tonic.
- Drink 1 cup daily to support reproductive health and improve circulation.
- Store in the refrigerator for up to 2 days if making in advance. Reheat as needed.

Prostate Health Herbal Infusion

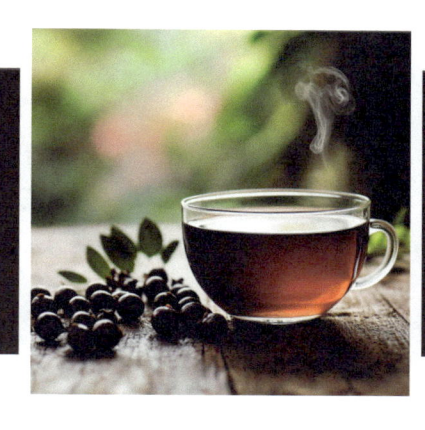

This infusion is made with saw palmetto, a powerful herb traditionally used to support prostate health. It is commonly used for reducing symptoms of benign prostatic hyperplasia (BPH) and may help improve urinary function in men. This soothing herbal infusion can be a natural addition to a wellness routine for maintaining prostate health.

Ingredients:

- Saw Palmetto Berries (1 tablespoon, dried): Saw palmetto is well-known for its role in supporting prostate health, particularly for relieving symptoms associated with an enlarged prostate.
- Water (1 cup): To make the infusion.

Instructions:

1. Add the saw palmetto berries to a cup of hot water.
2. Steep for 10-15 minutes.
3. Strain the herbs out and enjoy the infusion.
- Drink 1 cup daily to support prostate health and maintain urinary function.
- Store in the refrigerator for up to 2 days. Reheat as needed.

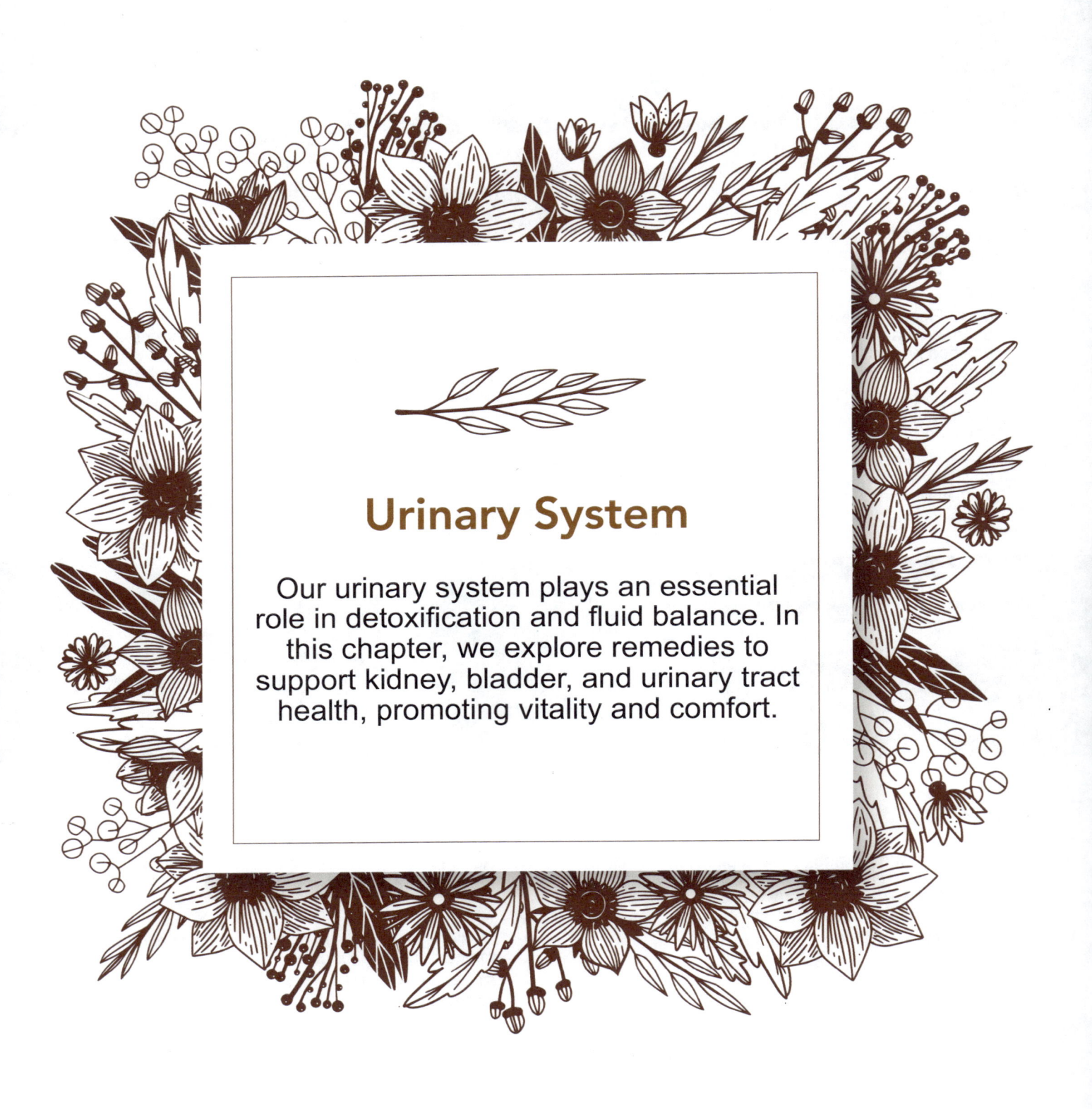

Urinary System

Our urinary system plays an essential role in detoxification and fluid balance. In this chapter, we explore remedies to support kidney, bladder, and urinary tract health, promoting vitality and comfort.

Soothing Corn Silk Tea

Corn silk tea has been traditionally used to support urinary health, providing relief from bladder discomfort and promoting prostate health. The soothing properties of corn silk help reduce inflammation and irritation in the urinary tract while promoting healthy urine flow.

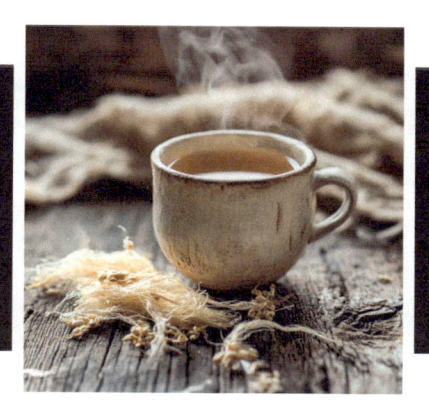

Ingredients:

- Corn Silk (1 tablespoon, dried): Known for its ability to support bladder and urinary tract health, corn silk also helps ease discomfort associated with prostate issues.
- Water (1 cup): To brew the tea.

Instructions:

1. Boil water and pour over dried corn silk in a teapot or cup.
2. Let it steep for 10-15 minutes.
3. Strain the herbs out and drink.

- Sip the tea once or twice a day to help soothe bladder discomfort and support prostate health.
- Best consumed fresh. Store any leftovers in the fridge for up to 1 day and reheat before drinking.

UTI-Fighting Herbal Tea Blend

This herbal blend targets urinary tract infections (UTIs) and helps soothe the discomfort caused by inflammation. The combination of herbs has natural antimicrobial properties that can support the body's ability to fight infections and promote a healthy urinary system.

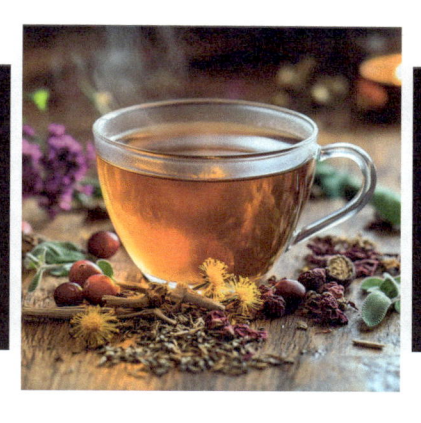

Ingredients:

- Uva Ursi (1 tablespoon, dried): Known for its strong antimicrobial properties, Uva Ursi helps to fight bacterial infections in the urinary tract.
- Cranberry (1 tablespoon, dried): Cranberries are rich in antioxidants and help prevent bacteria from adhering to the urinary tract walls.
- Dandelion Root (1 tablespoon, dried): Supports kidney and liver function and acts as a diuretic to help flush out bacteria from the urinary tract.
- Echinacea (1 teaspoon, dried): Known for its immune-boosting properties, Echinacea supports the body in fighting infections.
- Water (1 cup): For brewing the tea.

Instructions:

1. Boil water and pour over the dried herbs in a teapot or cup.
2. Let it steep for 10-15 minutes.
3. Strain the herbs out and drink.

- Drink 1-2 cups per day to support urinary tract health and help fight infection.
- Consume freshly made tea. You can store leftovers in the fridge for up to 1 day and reheat before drinking.

Cranberry Hibiscus Detox Tea

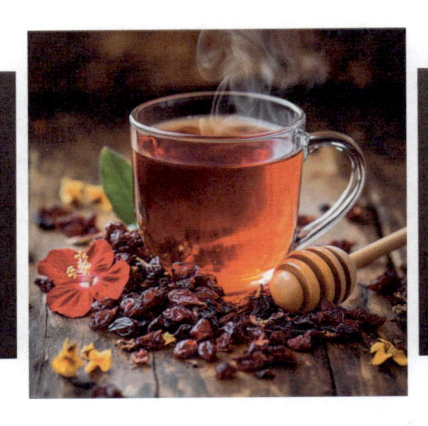

This vibrant, tangy tea is a perfect herbal remedy to support urinary health. The combination of cranberry and hibiscus offers natural benefits for preventing urinary tract infections and promoting bladder health. Cranberry is widely recognized for its ability to prevent bacterial adhesion in the urinary tract, while hibiscus provides soothing properties and supports kidney function.

Ingredients:

- Cranberry (1 tablespoon, dried or fresh): Known for its ability to prevent UTIs by inhibiting bacteria from sticking to the bladder wall.
- Hibiscus Flowers (1 tablespoon, dried): Rich in antioxidants, hibiscus can help maintain kidney health and soothe the urinary system.
- Honey (optional, 1 teaspoon): Adds sweetness and offers additional antibacterial benefits.
- Water (2 cups): For infusing the herbs.

Instructions:

1. Combine cranberry and hibiscus flowers in a teapot or heatproof jar.
2. Pour boiling water over the herbs and let them steep for 10-15 minutes.
3. Strain the tea and stir in honey, if desired.

- Drink 1-2 cups daily, especially during or after a UTI or for regular urinary system support.
- This tea is best enjoyed fresh. If storing, refrigerate for up to 1-2 days and reheat as needed.

Parsley Detox & Urinary Health Tea

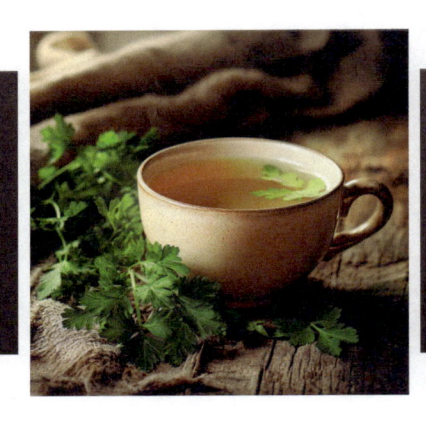

Parsley is not only a popular herb used for culinary purposes, but it also offers natural diuretic properties, making it beneficial for supporting urinary tract health and relieving inflammation. It helps flush excess fluids from the body, reduces swelling, and provides antioxidants that promote overall kidney and bladder health.

Ingredients:

- Parsley (1 tablespoon, dried or fresh): Known for its anti-inflammatory properties and ability to reduce swelling in the urinary tract, parsley also promotes detoxification and helps prevent infections.
- Water (2 cups): Used to infuse the herbs.

Instructions:

1. Place parsley in a heatproof jar or teapot.
2. Pour boiling water over the parsley and let it steep for 10-15 minutes.
3. Strain the tea to remove the herbs.

- Drink 1-2 cups daily, especially if experiencing inflammation or discomfort in the urinary tract.
- This tea is best consumed fresh. If you need to store it, keep it refrigerated for up to 1-2 days and reheat before drinking.

Kidney Cleanse Elixir

This kidney elixir is crafted to support kidney function and promote urinary tract health. The herbs in this blend are known for their diuretic properties, which help flush out toxins, promote urine flow, and support the body's natural detoxification processes.

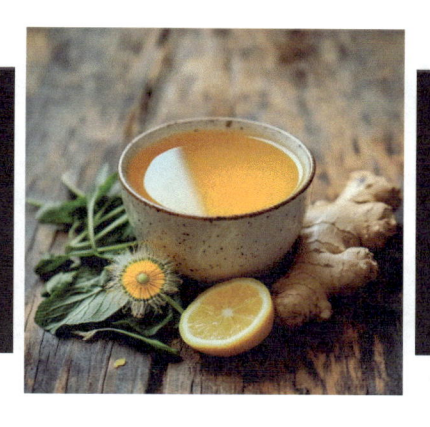

Ingredients:

- Dandelion Root (1 tspn, dried): Known for its diuretic properties, dandelion root helps cleanse the kidneys and supports overall urinary health.
- Nettle Leaf (1 tspn, dried): Supports kidney function, reduces inflammation, and promotes urine flow.
- Ginger Root (1 tspn, fresh or powdered): Known for its anti-inflammatory properties, ginger helps stimulate circulation and supports kidney health.
- Lemon Juice (juice of 1 lemon): Rich in antioxidants and vitamin C, lemon helps cleanse the kidneys and boosts detoxification.
- Honey (1 tspn): Adds natural sweetness while providing soothing and anti-inflammatory benefits.

Instructions:

1. Combine dandelion root, nettle leaf, and ginger in a heatproof jar or teapot.
2. Pour 2 cups of boiling water over the herbs and let it steep for 10-15 minutes.
3. Strain the herbs and stir in lemon juice and honey.

- Drink 1 cup of this elixir daily to support kidney function and urinary health.
- Best consumed fresh. You can store the elixir in the refrigerator for up to 1-2 days if needed. Always reheat before drinking.

Kidney Detox Juice

This refreshing juice is crafted to help cleanse and detoxify the kidneys while promoting urinary health. The combination of hydrating fruits and kidney-supporting herbs can help flush out toxins and maintain proper kidney function.

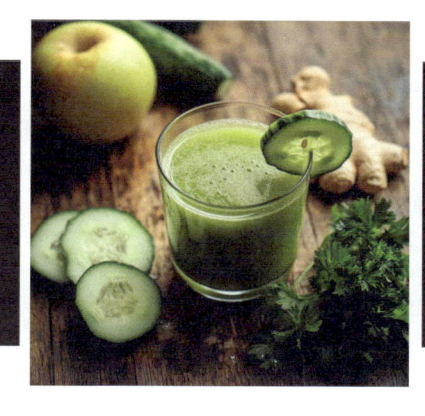

Ingredients:

- Cucumber (1/2 cucumber): A natural diuretic that helps hydrate the kidneys and flush out toxins.
- Lemon (juice of 1 lemon): Rich in antioxidants and vitamin C, which aids in detoxification and supports kidney health.
- Apple (1 medium): Packed with fiber and antioxidants, apple helps improve kidney function and supports detox.
- Parsley (1 tablespoon, fresh): Known for its diuretic properties, parsley helps stimulate urine production and flushes out waste.
- Ginger (1-inch piece, fresh): Supports circulation and has anti-inflammatory properties that help the kidneys function better.
- Water (1 cup): To mix and hydrate.

Instructions:

1. Add cucumber, apple, parsley, and ginger to a blender.
2. Squeeze in the lemon juice and add water.
3. Blend until smooth and strain if necessary.
- Drink this juice in the morning or after meals to support kidney detox and urinary health.
- Best consumed fresh. If stored, refrigerate for up to 1 day and re-blend before drinking.

Pumpkin Seed Bladder Support Tincture

Pumpkin seeds are known to support urinary health, particularly for those suffering from an overactive bladder. Rich in essential fatty acids, zinc, and antioxidants, pumpkin seeds help strengthen bladder muscles, reduce urinary urgency, and support the overall health of the urinary system.

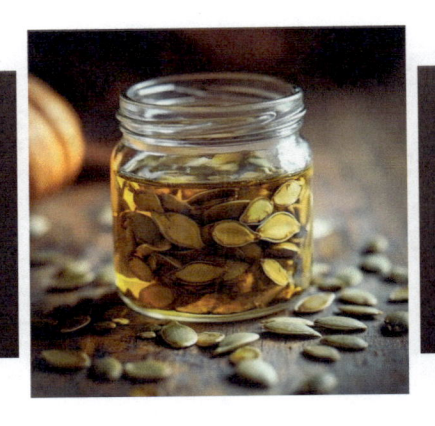

Ingredients:

- Pumpkin Seeds (1/4 cup, dried): Rich in zinc and fatty acids, pumpkin seeds help promote healthy bladder function and reduce urinary urgency.
- Vegetable Glycerin (1 cup): Used to create an alcohol-free tincture, making it gentle and safe for regular use.

Instructions:

1. Place the dried pumpkin seeds in a glass jar.
2. Pour the vegetable glycerin over the seeds, ensuring they are fully submerged.
3. Seal the jar tightly and let it sit in a cool, dark place for 2-4 weeks, shaking it once a day.
4. After the steeping period, strain out the seeds using a fine mesh strainer or cheesecloth.

- Take 1-2 dropperfuls in water, up to three times a day, especially during periods of bladder discomfort.
- Store in a cool, dark place for up to one year. Make a fresh batch as needed.

Apothecary Care & Storage Tips

Proper care and storage are essential for preserving the potency and freshness of your homemade remedies. With the right setup, your apothecary can remain a reliable, well-organized resource for months or even years. Here's a practical guide to organizing, storing, and extending the shelf life of your natural remedies.

Organizing Your Apothecary

- **Categorize by Type or Use:** Group items based on type (e.g., dried herbs, tinctures, essential oils) or intended use (e.g., sleep aids, immunity boosters, skincare). This makes it easier to find what you need without rummaging.

- **Label Everything Clearly:** Use durable labels with the name of the remedy, date of preparation, and any key ingredients. This helps you keep track of freshness and identify ingredients quickly.

- **Designate Storage Areas:** Create separate sections or shelves for different items (e.g., oils on one shelf, teas on another). This keeps everything orderly and minimizes the risk of cross-contamination.

Storing Remedies

- **Glass Containers:** Use airtight glass jars and bottles for dried herbs, tinctures, and oils. Glass preserves the freshness of remedies and doesn't leach chemicals like plastic can.

- **Dark Glass for Essential Oils and Tinctures:** Essential oils and some tinctures are sensitive to light, so amber or cobalt glass bottles are ideal for blocking harmful UV rays.

- **Keep Away from Heat and Light:** Store your remedies in a cool, dark place like a cabinet or pantry. Exposure to heat and light can degrade the active compounds in many ingredients, reducing their effectiveness.

- **Avoid Humidity:** Dried herbs are particularly sensitive to moisture. Store them in a dry area, ideally with silica packets or a small muslin bag of rice to absorb any extra humidity.

Maintaining Freshness

1. Rotate Stock Regularly: Use remedies in the order they were made to ensure that older items are used up first. This practice minimizes waste and helps maintain freshness.

2. Check Expiration Dates: While natural remedies don't often come with standard expiration dates, you can estimate shelf life based on the type of product:

- **Dried Herbs:** About 6–12 months. Watch for color or scent fading, which signals a loss of potency.

- **Tinctures:** 2–5 years, if alcohol-based. Vinegar-based tinctures last around a year.

- **Oils and Salves:** 1–2 years, depending on ingredients. Signs of rancidity include a change in smell or consistency.

- **Avoid Touching with Bare Hands:** For dried herbs and powdered ingredients, use clean utensils to prevent contamination. Oils from your hands can degrade the quality of some ingredients.

- **Refrigerate When Needed:** Certain items, like fresh aloe vera gel or some homemade creams, benefit from refrigeration to stay fresh longer. Always check if refrigeration is recommended for specific recipes.

- **Check Regularly for Mold or Rancidity:** Inspect stored items every few months to ensure there's no spoilage, mold, or off smells. Discard anything that seems questionable.

Proper Usage and Dosage

Herbal remedies can be highly effective, but using them properly is essential for safety and effectiveness. Here are key guidelines to follow:

- **Consult a Healthcare Provider:** Always check with a healthcare provider, especially if you have health conditions or take medications, to ensure there are no interactions.

- **Research the Herb:** Learn about the specific herb, its benefits, and possible side effects before use.

- **Start with Small Doses:** Begin with a small amount to see how your body reacts and gradually increase the dosage if needed.

- **Follow Recommended Dosages:** Stick to the recommended dosages provided by manufacturers or a healthcare professional.

- **Understand Different Forms:** Herbs come in various forms (teas, tinctures, oils, etc.), and each form may have different potency.

- **Be Aware of Side Effects:** Watch for any adverse reactions, such as digestive upset or allergic responses. Discontinue use if necessary.

- **Avoid Self-Medicating for Serious Conditions:** Herbal remedies are helpful for mild issues but should not replace medical care for serious conditions.

- **Store Properly:** Keep herbs in a cool, dry place to maintain their potency and avoid contamination.

By following these guidelines, you can ensure the safe and effective use of herbal remedies, tapping into the healing power of nature while protecting your health.

Side Effects and Allergies

Herbal remedies are generally safe but can cause side effects or allergic reactions. Here's what to watch for:

- **Common Side Effects:** Herbs can cause mild issues like digestive upset, headaches, or dizziness. If any symptoms occur, reduce the dose or stop use and consult a healthcare provider.

- **Allergic Reactions:** Some people may be allergic to certain herbs, causing rashes, itching, swelling, or difficulty breathing. Discontinue use and seek medical attention if these occur.

- **Drug Interactions:** Herbs can interact with medications, affecting their effectiveness or causing harmful reactions. Always check with a healthcare provider if you're on medication.

- **Toxicity:** Certain herbs can be toxic in large amounts. Always follow recommended dosages and avoid overuse.

- **Pregnancy and Breastfeeding:** Some herbs may not be safe during pregnancy or breastfeeding. Consult your healthcare provider before use.

Always start with small doses, be aware of potential reactions, and consult a healthcare provider for guidance.

Made in the USA
Columbia, SC
27 December 2024

50646156R00072